FEEDING
YOUR CHILD
The
Brazelton Way

also by T. Berry Brazelton, M.D.

On Becoming a Family
The Growth of Attachment Before and After Birth

Infants and Mothers
Differences in Development

Toddlers and Parents
Declaration of Independence

Doctor and Child

To Listen to a Child
Understanding the Normal Problems of Growing Up

Working and Caring

What Every Baby Knows

Families, Crisis, and Caring

Touchpoints
Your Child's Emotional and Behavioral Development

Going to the Doctor

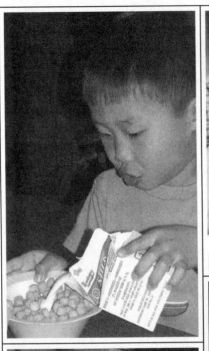
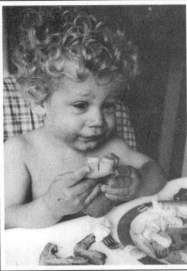
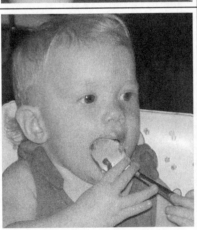
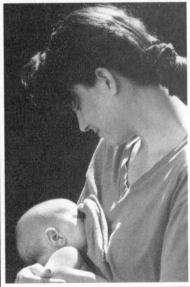

FEEDING YOUR CHILD
The
Brazelton Way

T. Berry Brazelton, M.D.
Joshua D. Sparrow, M.D.

A Merloyd Lawrence Book

DA CAPO PRESS
A Member of the Perseus Books Group

PHOTO CREDITS

Photographs on pages 12, 100 and title page [upper right] are by Janice Fullman

Photographs on page xvi and title page [lower right] are by Dorothy Littell Greco

Photographs on title page [upper and lower left] are by Marilyn Nolt

Text design by Trish Wilkinson

Set in 11-point Adobe Garamond by the Perseus Books Group

Cataloging-in-Publication data for this book is available from the Library of Congress.

First Da Capo Press edition 2004

ISBN 0-7382-0919-8

Published by Da Capo Press

A Member of the Perseus Books Group

http://www.dacapopress.com

Da Capo Press books are available at special discounts for bulk purchases in the U.S. by corporations, institutions, and other organizations. For more information, please contact the Special Markets Department at the Perseus Books Group, 11 Cambridge Center, Cambridge, MA 02142, or call (800) 255-1514 or (617) 252-5298, or e-mail specialmarkets@perseusbooks.com.

1 2 3 4 5 6 7 8 9—08 07 06 05 04

To the children and parents
who have taught us so much through the years

Contents

Preface

Ever since I wrote the first *Touchpoints* book, published in 1991, I have been asked by parents and professionals all over the country to write some short, easy-to-read books on the common challenges that parents face as they raise their children. Among the most common are crying, discipline, sleep, toilet training, and feeding.

In my 50 years of pediatric practice, families have taught me that problems in these areas often arise predictably as a child develops. In these short books I have tried to address the problems that parents are bound to encounter as their children regress just before they make their next developmental leap. Each book describes these "touchpoints" so that parents can better understand their child's behavior. Each also offers practical suggestions on how parents can help their child master the challenges and get back on track.

In general, these books focus on the concerns of the first six years of life, although occasionally older children's issues are referred to. In the final chapters, special problems are discussed.

These short books are not intended to cover such topics exhaustively. Instead, we hope that these books will serve as easy-to-use guides for parents to turn to as they face their child's growing pains, the "touchpoints" that inevitably arise as children and parents navigate these common and predictable childhood issues. For parents who want more information, references are provided for the topics covered.

As with *Touchpoints Three to Six,* I have invited Joshua Sparrow, M.D., to co-author these books with me, to add his perspective to mine. Although difficulties such as food refusal, weaning problems, and chaotic mealtimes are common and predictable, they make great demands on parents. These kinds of problems are, for the most part, temporary and not serious, yet without support and understanding, they can overwhelm a family and send a child's development seriously off course. We do not want to load parents down with advice that stops them from following their instincts, but instead to offer them the support they may need to understand their child and reaffirm their own expertise. It is our hope that the straightforward information provided in these books will help prevent those unnecessary derailments and provide reassurance for parents in times of uncertainty, so that the excitement and joy of helping a child grow can be rekindled.

Acknowledgments

We would like to thank parents across the country for having first urged us to write these concise, accessible books on topics of the utmost importance to them; without their vision, the books might never have been written. Thanks also go to Geoffrey Canada, Marilyn Josephs and the Baby College staff, Bart and Karen Lawson, David Saltzman, and Caressa Singleton for their unwavering support for our work—and from whom we have learned so much. Susan Frates, R.D., deserves special recognition for her careful review of our manuscript and her invaluable suggestions. As always, we would like to thank our editor, Merloyd Lawrence, for her wisdom and guidance. Finally, we wish to express our gratitude to our families, not only for their encouragement and patience, but for the lessons they have taught us that we have sought to impart in this book.

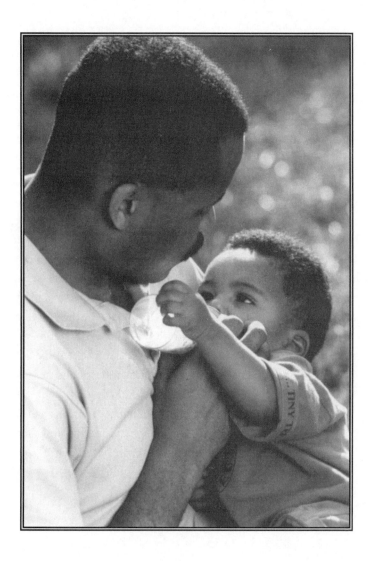

CHAPTER 1

A Parent's First Job

Feeding a child is a sacred mission for a parent. From the first stirring of the baby in the womb, a parent-to-be feels: "This will be my new life. It will be up to me to assure that my baby grows and thrives. Feeding her well will be my job—one part of all that responsibility." This new role may begin to feel like a challenge even before the child is born. After birth, although feeding may lead to more worries, it is more likely to be a source of great pleasure—from the very first feeding—for parents and baby.

Touchpoints—A Predictable Path for Development

The steps along the path taken by dedicated, responsible parents and their child are predictable ones. There are times when the child will be difficult to feed. These predictable hurdles, which I call "touchpoints," often precede a new burst of independence in the child.

When a strong-willed child is eager for more participation in feeding—holding the bottle, sippie cup, or spoon or flinging

1

hunks of food from the high chair—parents can feel challenged. These touchpoints occur as a child is ready to take on a larger role in caring for herself. Parents sense the child's pulling away. They may try to regain control, lest they lose the child they have learned to understand. But parents can also learn to let go and feel proud of their child's new resourcefulness. When they do, feeding will again become a source of pleasure and a special time for being together.

I call these times of change touchpoints because I have found that passionate parents can reevaluate their role if I can reach out to them at the right time with the information they need—revealing the child's struggle as an important one for her future development. We hope you can use Chapter Two, "The Touchpoints of Feeding," to help you watch for the conflict between your child's goals for independence and yours for "getting her fed properly." As you learn to prepare yourself for these times, you'll find it easier to plan your child's meals, and encourage her participation in them.

Chapter Three, "Feeding Challenges and Opportunities," addresses common problems that arise as children learn to eat, and parents learn to feed them, in the first years. As you can see, this book is not meant to be an exhaustive guide to pediatric nutrition or gastrointestinal illness. While pointing out some basics, it focuses on the behavior and psychological issues that accompany feeding, from the beginning of life through the early years. Specialized questions, for example, about food additives, allergies, or digestive disorders can be pursued through the books and resources in the bibliography.

"Ghosts from the Nursery"

As a baby grows, a parent's responsibility to nurture can seem even greater. No wonder a parent can find it difficult to turn feeding over to the child as the child fights for independence in making her own choices. My own mother, a sensitive and worthy lady, could not let my younger brother learn to feed himself on his own. My memories of meals when we were little are of her cajoling, singing, and poking bits of food at him for two hours at each meal. He, in turn, was in control. His jaw muscles bulged as they held his mouth shut. His eyes were rather merry as he led my mother through the two-hour battle. "Please, just one bite!" she would plead, over and over, to no avail.

This experience became a "ghost" in my own nursery, an expression that child expert Selma Fraiberg coined to describe the effects of certain childhood memories on adult behavior. It helped set my future. I eventually determined to become a physician who could turn parents' passion toward positive approaches to child rearing, especially in the area of feeding. Many parents discover their own "ghosts," childhood memories about being fed, as they accompany their own child through the touchpoints of feeding.

By the end of the first year, for example, control over choice and quantity of food must become the child's. Many parents find it hard to turn that job over to the child. However, no parent can successfully force a child to eat: a battle over food is one the parent is sure to lose. Parents can only present the child with healthy choices.

Feeding oneself and making one's own choices is a necessary goal for any young child. Parents will have to learn to give up the delicious sensation of the baby nursing in their arms and to enjoy instead the mealtime company of a 1-year-old who is more interested in testing out gravity with her food than she is in putting it in her mouth. Ultimately, though, enjoying the pleasure of being together that goes along with mealtimes will be the most effective way for parents to support the child's development of healthy eating habits.

When parents struggle with a child over food—what to eat and how much—the child's hunger seems to lose its importance. Hunger is a basic instinct, controlled by a fairly primitive part of the brain. However, more complex parts of a child's brain are set in motion and can override hunger. This occurs, for example, when a child begins to wonder, "Do I have to eat this because my mother says I do? Can she make me?" When there's a chance for a struggle, a child's hunger may not be enough to push a child to eat. If there is turmoil over food between parent and child, food loses its primary meaning—as a necessity for health and a source of comfort and pleasure.

Sometimes such struggles arise from a parents' "ghosts," sometimes from limitations in the baby or young child's ability to suck, swallow, coordinate chewing movements, keep food down, and so on. Often these factors work together. Struggles over food are always passionate. Parents everywhere know that food is as necessary to survival as air, and they care deeply about their child's survival and growth. Children, for their part, have strong preferences from an early age. Cultural traditions are also an important part of a parent's passion.

A Parent's Passion

Parents' commitment to feed their children and to protect them from malnutrition is powerful. This became clear to me in a study we did of a malnourished group of Mayan Indians in Guatemala in 1978. Pregnant women were subsisting on 1,200–1,400 calories a day, even though more than 2,000 calories per day (exact amounts vary depending on height, activity level, and other factors) would be necessary for adequate nourishment of the developing fetus's brain.

We tried to increase their diet to an adequate level. We offered these women a daily 1,000-calorie liquid supplement. They came into our local center each day to get the supplement, take it home, and then—use it to feed the rest of the family! Our special liquid supplement for these pregnant women never reached their fetuses. The mothers felt they must first feed their already born children. The sad result was a lower than expected IQ by the time these unborn babies reached school age.

When we finally recognized the obvious, that of course a mother would feed her children before feeding herself, we changed our tactics. We began to urge these well-meaning women to drink the supplement "in order to have smart babies." When they understood that they were not just taking this additional food for their own benefit, but instead for their unborn babies' well-being, they were willing to drink it themselves. How powerful is the maternal instinct to protect her offspring!

Brain Development
Begins Before Birth

The Guatemalan study also showed us the strong influences of poor nutrition on children's development. We learned that lower intelligence was all too likely if children were undernourished in the womb or in early infancy. At birth, babies who have been undernourished during pregnancy are already less responsive to nurturing. Mothers may then feed them "when they want it," often only three times a day for a lethargic baby, rather than the 6 to 8 feedings a day that well-fed newborns usually demand.

Even in a land of plenty, parents are just as passionate about their responsibility to ensure that their child is well nourished. In fact, our increased understanding about the effects of nutrition on health and early brain development can lead parents to put pressure on their children. This can interfere with pleasure in eating—the second most important motivator for children after hunger.

There is still much to be learned about nutrition. In the meantime, a child who learns to enjoy eating a wide variety of foods will receive the balance of nutrients that, as far as we know now, will best help her grow up healthy and strong. For a child to develop this kind of curiosity and flexibility about food, mealtimes need to be fun, relaxing, and a time for a family to enjoy being together. In this book we suggest ways to keep them that way.

Pressure from others, along with a parent's sense of duty, can get in the way. So can a child's struggles to eat independently. Parents need to be prepared for the touchpoints in which struggles are likely to arise. The goal must, of course, be for a child to feed herself independently and to *enjoy* eating enough of the right kinds of foods to help her grow and be healthy. Parents will want to take into account the child's temperament as well as the developmental challenges of each touchpoint, which we will explain in Chapter Two.

Temperament

Feeding a Quiet Child

A quiet, sensitive child may be on a different track from her peers. She may comply with being fed and continue to be compliant even during the usual times of conflict. For example, unlike other children her age, she may allow herself to be fed into the second year, apparently content to be a passive recipient. Then, all of a sudden, refusal! No longer will she put up with being fed. Passive resistance may be her response.

Her refusal to be fed is a warning to her parents to pull back and let her try feeding herself. Since she has not had experience with finger feeding or with utensils, her first attempts to feed herself may be clumsy. A big mess at every meal—food on her face, her clothes, the table, the floor, everywhere—will be the inescapable price for her earlier compliance.

Parents may even be thankful for the slobbery mess when it comes—a welcome relief from the initial food refusal of this phase of self-assertion! Patience with such a child will be the saving grace. Let her learn how to take over the job of feeding. Offer her only two bits at a time of an attractive finger food for each meal. Then ignore her struggle and leave it to her. Keep her company, but don't cajole during meals. If and when she downs the two bits, offer her two more at a time, until she starts smooshing them or launching them over the edge of her high chair. This means it's time to stop—until the next meal. Don't let her "graze" between meals. And for now, don't worry about a well-rounded diet. Remember that this previously compliant child is quickly learning the skills of self-feeding. It might have taken her several months longer to learn had she been less passive and started in with her attempts to take over her own feeding earlier. Be patient and follow her lead.

Feeding an Active Child

At the other end of the temperament spectrum is the active, constantly moving, curious-about-everything child. She is far more interested in sights, sounds, and rushing around than in food. A parent whose motive is to see that the child is well fed is bound to feel frustrated, even desperate. "Sit down in your seat," a worried parent will beg as the child climbs out of her high chair to hang teetering on the edge. The child looks up coyly, holding out one hand for a "cookie." Anything she can eat will do as long as at the same time she can clamber around the house, up and over furniture and into drawers to pull out clean clothes with grubby fingers.

Many parents of active children have asked me: "Should I feed her on the run? She'll never eat enough sitting down. She barely sits before she's gone. I wait until she's hungry, but she never is. I feel like I need to give her bits of food all through the day so that she'll get enough. What should I do?"

My advice has been:

1. Keep mealtimes a sacred time for the family to be together. Don't let the phone or other interruptions interfere.
2. When your child loses interest in sitting at the table—that's it. Put her down and let her know her meal is over. No grazing between meals. No more food until the next meal.
3. Make meals a fun time to be together—at least as much as is possible with a squirming, food-throwing toddler. Make meals as companionable as possible—you eat when she does. But if she doesn't, eat your own meal and let her know that you can chat and be together if she stays at the table. If she squirms to leave, put her down. But she'll have to wait for your attention until you're done. Eventually she'll learn to model on you.
4. No television at the table or promises of special sweet desserts to get her to sit and eat.
5. Be sure you let her feed herself. Never say, "Just one more bite." If you do, you'll be setting yourself up for testing.
6. Don't go to special trouble to cook her a special or exciting meal—your disappointment is likely to outweigh the

benefits. Instead, let your child know that "this is what we're having for dinner tonight." If she doesn't want it, she'll have to see if she likes the next meal any better.

7. Let her help with meals as soon as she is old enough to do even the smallest task, such as setting the table (start with the napkins only!), cleaning it with a sponge, and so on.

8. Have your child's pediatrician check her weight and growth, and ask her for supplements if necessary.

9. Above all, don't set meals up as a struggle or her high chair as a prison to keep her in.

Beyond Nutrition

Right from the first, feeding is an opportunity for intimacy. Parents find such satisfaction in being able to provide a child with what she needs and to enjoy with her the pleasure of eating. Mealtimes are opportunities for parents and child to relax and enjoy each other. If parents can manage their own feelings about their child's independence in this area, the child will look forward to meals, to eating the way the rest of the family do.

Table manners and attitudes toward mealtimes are learned in the fourth and fifth years as children model on their elders. Keep mealtimes pleasant. Use them as times for communication with each other. Save other times for difficult topics that need to be discussed. More than ever today, families under stress need the rituals of mealtimes to bring them together. Children need to share meals with the rest of the family, not with the television.

More Ghosts from the Nursery

Parents bring many kinds of childhood experiences with food to the table. As a young pediatrician, I would never have admitted it, but while I was recommending that parents eat with their children, I began to get a stomach ulcer from eating with my own. My stomach hurt after each meal. I found myself making comments that I'd never recommend to other parents: "Just eat one taste of that—you'll like it." My children would look up at me as if to say, "Why should I like it?" When they lagged behind at table, I would steal a bit off their plates, as if to spur them on to eat, "before Daddy stole their food."

They have never forgotten my foolish antics, and they have never understood why I cared so much about how much and what they ate. Fortunately, my stomach pains began to disappear when I became aware of the reason for my behavior—a ghost from my own nursery, the memory of my mother pushing my brother to eat. Although I escaped her pressure myself, it was in the air at our mealtimes.

As a result, I would advise parents to reevaluate their own experience when they find that they are getting uptight about what and how much their child is eating. "Ghosts" interfere with common sense and are more likely to affect your behavior if you're not aware of them. If you are aware of them, you can make choices. My grandchildren have given me a second chance. I do not steal food from my grandchildren's plates. Nor do I press their parents any longer to eat "a rounded diet." They do anyway.

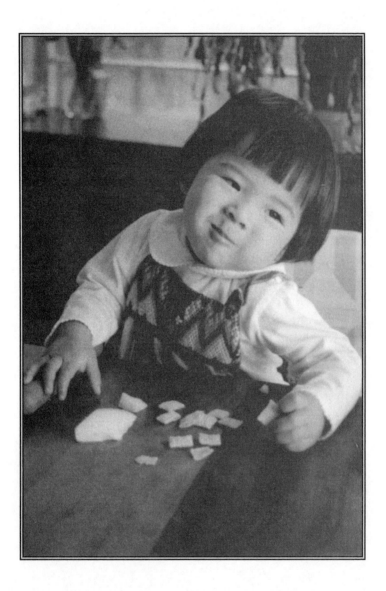

CHAPTER 2

The Touchpoints of Feeding

Breast or Bottle: Making the Choice

During the last 3 months of pregnancy, it is time to decide whether to breastfeed or bottle-feed. As a pediatrician, I like to have a prenatal visit with expectant parents during the seventh month of pregnancy. This is a good time to share such questions, because the process of birth and delivery are not yet looming large. Soon, though, they will be, and parents will have other concerns.

In this prenatal visit, I can get to know both parents without a baby between us. Each parent is likely to discuss his or her plans, wishes, and fears about becoming a parent. It can be a time for us to share their concerns and their hopes for the baby. All parents-to-be wonder, "How will I ever learn to be a parent? What kind of baby will I have?"

When I ask, "How do you plan to feed your baby?" it gives us a chance to discuss the decision to breastfeed or to use formula.

Benefits of Breastfeeding for the Baby

As a pediatrician, I am biased. The American Academy of Pediatrics recommends breastfeeding for 12 months. Among the reasons:

1. Breast milk is made for babies. Cow's milk is made for calves. While formulas today are as good as they can be and are fairly digestible, a certain number of babies will be allergic to cow's milk formula. I have never had a patient who was allergic to breast milk. A rare baby is sensitive to foods that the mother may eat and transmit in her breast milk. Usually these can be readily eliminated from her diet. But breast milk sensitivities are almost nonexistent. Cow's milk sensitivities may be difficult to detect initially. They may not show up as skin rashes or stomach upsets for several months. When a baby is allergic to cow's milk formula, it must be replaced with a substitute. (See *Milk and Milk Allergies* in Chapter Three.)

2. Breast milk provides the newborn with the mother's antibodies to protect the baby from infection. Colostrum, the cloudy liquid that precedes the breast milk by two or three days, is especially loaded with antibodies against infection. Breast milk is protective all through the period of breastfeeding, lowering the risk of ear infections, coughs, and colds. In fact, it also appears to protect babies against rashes and other signs of allergies.

3. You cannot overfeed your baby with breast milk alone—even if breastfed babies feed often and grow to appear "fat" in

the process. A baby who seems to fatten on breast milk is likely to lose unnecessary fat after weaning. A baby does need to be weighed periodically by his pediatrician to be sure that he is receiving enough nutrition and growing as he should. Then you can relax and enjoy the times for nursing together!

4. Breast milk provides a baby with the nutrients he needs most in the first year. It even provides some of the digestive enzymes a baby needs to handle them. Even when mothers are malnourished, the nutritional value of breast milk is protected by nature. But, of course, a mother's diet will influence the levels of certain vitamins and minerals in breast milk.

Women who are breastfeeding should check with their doctors before taking medications, as some can pass from a mother's bloodstream into her breast milk.

A breastfeeding mother will need to drink enough fluids—2 or 3 quarts per day. She will also need to add at least 300 calories per day to the Recommended Dietary Allowances. (This can be done by adding one small meal a day, including a fruit, one vegetable, a piece of bread, a helping of meat or other high protein food such as cheese, nuts, or peanut butter, and two glasses of milk or other dairy products. These can be split up across the day instead, as added snacks. This is not the time for dieting!) But supplements will be important for some women who breastfeed. Women who are vegetarians should take a supplement with iron and vitamin B_{12}. Also, women who are unable to eat a balanced diet on a regular basis would do well to take a multivitamin supplement with iron while breastfeeding. Whether breastfeeding or not, women should continue taking iron supplements after delivery to rebuild their own iron stores.

Recently the American Academy of Pediatrics recommended a total minimum daily intake of 200 International Units of vitamin D for all infants, beginning within the first 2 months of life and continuing through childhood and adolescence. Once breastfed infants have been weaned and are taking in at least a pint of vitamin D–fortified milk or formula per day, they will not need supplements. Some infants will need iron supplements as well. Ask your baby's pediatrician about these supplements. Be careful, because your baby will need just the right amount. Too much vitamin D or iron can be dangerous!

For Bottle-Feeding

Many women who can't breastfeed feel guilty. But they needn't. There are many other ways to establish the same kind of closeness with bottle-feeding that they had hoped to experience with breastfeeding.

Some mothers are unable to breastfeed for medical reasons. Some medical obstacles to breastfeeding—such as inverted nipples, inadequate breast milk production, and nipple infections, can often be overcome, often with the assistance of a lactation consultant. (See, for example, La Leche League under *Resources*.) Sometimes mothers must take medications that can get through to their breast milk (most medications do) and could be dangerous for their babies. Mothers infected with HIV must not breastfeed, as their milk can transmit the virus to their babies.

Although my bias is for breastfeeding when it is possible, I have listened to the reasons against it that some mothers offer when they decide to bottle-feed their baby-to-be. Here are some of them and my responses.

1. Some mothers do not want to be at the mercy of feeding around the clock. They may prefer to use a bottle so that fathers and others can feed the baby too. They fear that if they breastfeed, no one else will be able to help out with feedings. This is not entirely true, as many breastfed babies will take a bottle too, if it's offered early (that is, before 3 weeks of age). One bottle a day need not interfere with a mother's milk production. When a mother is breastfeeding, I would recommend that a new father or a grandmother start offering one bottle a day (especially in the middle of the night!) by about 3 weeks, but only after the mother's breast milk has become plentiful. Starting a bottle sooner, or giving too much formula, may prevent a mother from developing a good supply of milk. But waiting too long can lead to a "breast-only" baby.

2. Some mothers may not feel comfortable with breastfeeding. For some, breastfeeding may not fit with the way they think about their bodies. Perhaps some were bottle-fed themselves as infants. For some, breastfeeding might seem too invasive. Many women feel embarrassed to have to feed without privacy. All of these reasons deserve respect. Sometimes, with support rather than badgering, women with concerns like these may reconsider their decision.

3. The wait for breast milk can be 4 to 5 days with the first baby. Meanwhile, it may be difficult to get the baby to suckle if the nipples are inverted or flattened. But a new mother can find help, such as a lactation expert. A lactation consultant can help her get her baby to awaken enough to suckle and to accept her nipple. Meanwhile, frequent stimulation of the nipple encourages production of breast milk.

4. With a bottle, you can see how much milk the baby is getting. This can be reassuring for a new, anxious parent. But if a breastfed baby is urinating about every four hours this is a sign that he's getting enough. When your doctor weighs and measures him at each routine visit and finds him to be growing well, then you can be sure he is getting enough milk.

5. Mothers who must go back to work are concerned about the job of pumping at work every 3–4 hours, of saving milk to bring home, and of leaving the baby with an adequate supply. They may also be especially concerned about the inconvenience of leaking milk as they struggle to balance work and motherhood. However, more companies are offering private areas for new mothers, and pumping and saving milk has become a successful routine for many mothers.

6. Many working mothers have confided in me that they are already grieving in pregnancy about having to leave their baby with someone else. They are afraid that breastfeeding will make them feel too close, and the baby too dependent.

When it is time to leave their baby with someone else, they fear that the grief will be even more excruciating. I try to show them that this closeness gives the baby a wonderful start, and that coming home to breastfeed can be a special time to feel close again each day. Of course, as a society we must do more to provide support—through daycare, parental leave, and corporate backing—for mothers who want to breastfeed.

7. Although science has not yet been able to produce a formula matching breast milk's virtues, some mothers think of breastfeeding as backwards or old-fashioned. Sadly, these views—spread with formula marketing—seem to have taken hold in the very parts of the world where women can't always afford to buy formula and where limited medical care makes breast milk's unique protection against infection even more important. Such promotion must be balanced by education about breastfeeding, as the American Academy of Pediatrics and groups such as La Leche League have done admirably.

The Most Important Ingredient

Whether breastfeeding or bottle-feeding, the bonding that comes with each feeding is the most important ingredient. Although every new mother will have several days of waiting and of struggling to get the baby to "learn" how to breastfeed, it can be so rewarding when it is finally successful. The same closeness and bonding can and must go on when formula is used.

Breastfeeding's Benefits for a Mother's Body

1. When your baby suckles, your hormones (oxytocin) help your uterus contract. The slightly uncomfortable pains that accompany the contraction last only 2–3 days, but they are a sign that your uterus is shrinking back to its normal size.
2. This hormone will also help reduce your postpartum bleeding.
3. Breastfeeding can act as a natural contraceptive, nature's way of helping to space out births. But be careful—it's not 100 percent effective! Even if you have not started to menstruate again, you still may ovulate and could get pregnant again. Too many breastfeeding mothers get pregnant again before they're ready.
4. Studies have shown that breastfeeding even reduces the later risk of breast cancer.

Before your baby is born, choose a comfortable rocking chair. You will want to sit with him to rouse him to a quick alert state in which he is ready to suckle. You'll soon be singing to him or talking quietly to him. Breastfeeding and bottle-feeding are ready opportunities for a mother and baby to feel close. A baby nurses in a suck-suck-suck pattern when he is initially fed. After several minutes, when he's no longer so hungry, the baby's nursing rhythm changes to a suck-suck-suck-pause, suck-suck-suck-pause pattern. This is repeated every minute or so. Dr. Kenneth Kaye and I noticed that a parent would jiggle or stir up the baby at the pauses. She might look down to say,

"Keep going." If the baby looked up at her, she'd say, "Love, keep feeding. You are just great!"

When we asked the mother why she jiggled or talked to him, she'd say, "I want him to keep eating. When he pauses, I'm afraid he'll stop." We timed the length of pauses when mothers stimulated their babies to start sucking again, and compared these with the pauses when they instead left it to the infants to start up on their own. To our surprise, when the mothers left the babies to start sucking again on their own, the pauses were shorter than when they responded to the babies' pauses with their own efforts to get the babies going again.

We concluded that when mothers interacted with their babies in these ways, the babies actually put off sucking and prolonged the pauses so that they could take in and respond to their mothers' communications with them. What an important way to foster closeness and responsiveness! Breastfeeding, a baby's sucking patterns, and a mother's responses all seem to be nature's ways of encouraging mother and baby to get to know one another. Feeding is a time for communication and learning each other's rhythms. The suck-suck-suck-pause pattern also occurs with bottle-feeding as an opportunity for this rewarding interaction.

Feeding the Baby Before Birth

From the beginning of pregnancy, every mother-to-be has a chance at the thrill of feeling her unborn baby growing inside her and the satisfaction of knowing that she is doing everything she can to nourish the fetus right from the first. Of course, morning sickness can make this more difficult, especially during the first 3 months. Many pregnant women, though, find that dry crackers, flat soda, grapefruit juice, and other traditional remedies help. Often, the worst of the nausea subsides by the end of the first trimester.

In addition to eating a healthy and well-balanced diet, pregnant women will want to be sure to take the vitamins and minerals prescribed at their prenatal care visits. Women need more calories and more of certain vitamins and minerals during pregnancy, when they are eating for two. Folic acid, for example, will protect your baby from certain birth defects, but you'll need more than when you're not pregnant. Iron protects mother and fetus against iron deficiency anemia. Taking 50 percent more calcium than what women who are not pregnant need will keep your bones strong while your baby's bones are growing. Check with your doctor about your supplements, because too much iron, calcium, and certain vitamins can be harmful. At each prenatal care visit, your doctor or nurse–midwife will help you be sure that your diet, vitamin and mineral supplements, and weight gain are the best they can be for your baby-to-be's healthy development inside of you.

It is important to avoid alcohol and tobacco, as well as exposure to high levels of lead, during pregnancy. Alcohol, tobacco, and lead can damage the unborn baby's developing brain. Tobacco also interferes with the transfer of food through the placenta from mother to fetus, increasing the risk of low birth weight. If you need help to stop smoking or drinking alcohol, be sure to ask your doctor. You deserve help, not judgment, especially at this important time.

A Father's Role

A father is likely to feel left out in this discussion of feeding. But of course he should be included. New fathers are both relieved and saddened by their wives' overpowering importance to the baby. Many fathers will withdraw from responsibility as a reaction to this new imbalance. Others may become more protective of their wives in an effort to see that the pregnancy goes well for the baby-to-be.

Any father deserves to be assured that he can help support the new mother in getting the feedings going. He can be urged to be present when the lactation consultant coaches the mother on helping her new baby suckle successfully. Also, as mentioned earlier, if a mother decides to breastfeed, I encourage the father to feed the baby a bottle no more than once a day by the third week. (See *Bibliography* for useful guides to a healthy pregnancy.)

The New Baby

Breastfeeding in the First Weeks

As you cuddle your newborn next to your breasts, his arms contained by yours, he may rouse to open his eyes. He may squint at first. He has always seen light dimly, through the filters of the womb. This new, bright light is overwhelming. As he feels your body against his, he quiets down. His hand grasps your finger.

He's likely to pull it up to his mouth. Let him suck on it. (Be sure it is washed, with the nail facing down in his mouth.) He is trying to learn how to suck. He needs practice. As you insert a finger you can feel the three parts of his sucking:

1. The soft chomping of the front of his tongue on your finger against the roof of his mouth
2. The soft rhythmic lapping of the back of his tongue
3. The suction of his throat and esophagus as he tries to pull nourishment out of your finger

By attending carefully, you can feel these three start off independently. Then, as they gather "experience," they begin to pull together. An effective pull is one where all three are coordinated in unison. Imagine being able to let him "learn" how to get the three elements of sucking to come together on your finger! He is preparing for the breast or bottle.

Feeding Position

In the first months of a baby's life, positioning for feeding is critical to success. (Later, he'll readjust his position—if he needs to—on his own.) First of all, make sure you are as comfortable as possible. Then, tilt him up at a 30 degree angle in your arms. Rock him gently from side to side to try to alert him gently. After all, he has just been through a pretty dramatic time—squished by uterine contractions, and squirming to get out of the birth canal. Even if he was born by cesarean section, he may first have been through enough labor to have awakened him to do his active part. Either way, he must now adapt to his new extrauterine environment—overly lit and overly noisy. How amazing that he can come to be alert at all! But if he can, he may be ready to try to suckle on your breast.

You may want an extra pillow to prop your baby on. Hold him in the crook of your arm, and trap one of his arms under yours. Use your hand to flatten out your breast, to keep the nipple protruding. Gently stroke his cheek next to your breast, and around the mouth on the side next to the breast. This will set off his rooting reflex. But don't stroke both of his cheeks. This will only confuse him. Be ready to offer him your nipple when he turns to it. Don't be too active, or you'll overwhelm him. A gentle, respectful approach is best.

Try to feed him in a quiet place. When he turns to the breast and opens his mouth, insert your flattened nipple and breast into his open mouth. If you can get your nipple into the back of his throat and to touch the base of his tongue, the sucking response will be at its best. Be sure he can breathe while he sucks by pressing down your breast with one finger so that he can breathe through his tiny nostrils. Gently rock and jiggle him a bit to keep him awake. Once he starts sucking, he will taste your colostrum. This should stimulate him to keep sucking.

Colostrum

Your milk won't come in for 4–5 days with your first baby. But the cloudy fluid that he will get, the colostrum, is very valuable. It is rich in antibodies and full of protein. As we said earlier, it protects the baby from many kinds of infection.

Does Breast Size Matter?

Mothers with small breasts often think they won't have enough milk (especially in the United States, where quantity and quality are often confused). They will. The breast is an amazing organ. It responds to demand. When a baby needs more, the breasts engorge more to meet his demand. Incredible!

Breast and Nipple Care

Painful breast swelling or engorgement can occur because of hormones that become active after birth as the breasts enlarge to produce milk. If the breasts are swollen and painful, use warm washcloths as compresses before nursing, and cool compresses between feedings. Help your baby latch on. As he suckles, the engorgement will decrease. After a few days, your breasts will adjust to meet your baby's needs. If you have severe pain, or fever, call your doctor.

Sore and cracked nipples can be a problem in the beginning. Massaging your nipples with a lanolin-containing cream during late pregnancy may prepare them. Once you've begun nursing, you can protect your nipples by spreading a little of your milk over them and then letting them air dry after each feeding. Sore nipples sometimes occur when a baby does not take in the entire nipple and area of darkened skin around it. Let him suck on your finger first. Then he'll approach your nipple more gently and suck more effectively.

If you get a sore crack in a nipple, call your doctor as soon as you can. She or he can give you a cream to protect the crack and help it heal. You may have to avoid nursing with that breast for a day or two, though you'll probably have to express milk from it to keep it from becoming painfully swollen. If any sore, reddened areas appear, let your doctor know right away. Redness, swelling, pain, and skin that is especially warm to the touch are all signs of infection. Breast infections or abscesses can be treated and cured before they are a problem—the sooner the better.

Breastfeeding—How Often?

At first, you will want to limit the time your baby suckles on each breast so that your nipple tissue can adjust and become stronger. Gently take him off after just a few minutes on each side. He will take in the most milk in these first minutes. Don't pull him off your breast forcibly, as this can hurt your nipple. Instead, put one finger in the side of his mouth to let air in, to break the suction before you take him off.

At first, it may be important to feed him often, even 12–14 times a day, for short periods only, to allow your nipples to toughen up slowly. Use both breasts at each feeding. This will also increase your milk supply. Gently express any milk he leaves after a feeding. Stop massaging when the breast stops squirting. Getting the breasts emptied helps them to make more milk. This way you'll be ready for the next feed, when he may be hungrier. His hunger may not be as regular as your milk production.

Gradually increase feedings to 5 minutes and then 10 minutes per side when your milk comes in, and up to 20 minutes over the next few weeks. Let your nipples air dry after feedings, and use soft pads in your bra.

A Successful Beginning

When you have overcome these initial hurdles, you and the baby will know each other more deeply. You'll both feel in rhythm with each other, and indescribably close. Your baby's sucking even stimulates the release of hormones in you that leave you with a sense of well-being unlike anything you've ever experienced. It's as if breastfeeding and its effect on your hormones were meant to help you recover from the exhaustion of delivery and to bond with your new baby.

When the baby starts sucking, you will feel the so-called letdown reflex as milk is "let down" to fill your breasts. The other breast may leak at the same time, especially at first. Use a towel or a pad to catch the leaking. You may even let milk down when you hear your baby cry. Demand usually determines your milk supply. The more your baby sucks, the more milk you supply. If you are getting worn out or depressed by too many feedings, consult your physician. She or he will weigh your baby to see whether the feedings are enough for him before advising you about when and how often to feed.

Breastfeeding should begin to be rewarding after the initial adjustments in the first weeks. You can begin to feel that you have made it! You can add your satisfaction with this major accomplishment to the natural pleasure of getting to know your baby so intimately. Each feeding becomes an opportunity to communicate and to fall in love all over again. You have given him, his brain, his bodily functions, such a marvelous beginning. The struggle is worth it!

Bottle Feeding in the First Weeks

Although the baby will miss out on the colostrum and the antibodies contained in breast milk, formulas today are adjusted to babies' needs. Certainly, you should consult your physician in choosing the right formula for your baby. The cow's milk (or soybean milk) will have been modified or processed extensively to make it more digestible. Vitamins and minerals are added. You can be sure that they will cover your baby's nutritional needs. (Evaporated milk formulas are no longer recommended.)

A bottle of formula can be prepared from powdered formula or canned liquid formula, ready to give in just a few minutes. Follow the instructions on the box or can for preparing it. Be sure to use the amount of water called for by the instructions so that your baby gets a balance of nutrients and water with each feed. Some mothers have used less water than the instructions advise, in order to make the formula stronger so the baby will gain weight more rapidly. *Don't.* The baby's immature kidneys cannot tolerate the extra load of too much protein and salts. They need the water to dilute the salts and protein break-down products and form urine to rid the body of waste. If too much water is mixed in with formula, your baby will feel full too soon and stop feeding before he's taken in all the nutrients he needs.

The instructions should also tell you how long your formula will keep once it is opened, and once prepared. An opened box of powdered formula will stay fresh for a month if covered. A can of liquid formula should also be covered once opened, but must be refrigerated, and discarded after 48 hours. Even when refrigerated, a bottle of prepared formula won't keep for more than a day. Be sure also to read expiration dates on formula cans and packages.

What water to use: If you can't count on your local water supply, you can buy sterilized water for making baby formula. You can boil tap water for 5 minutes if it is otherwise safe to drink—if it contains no lead or other known contaminants. Be sure to let it cool down before mixing it with formula, to avoid destroying nutrients. You don't need to sterilize your baby's bottles and nipples as long as you wash them with hot, soapy water and scrub them with a bottle brush. Rinse carefully.

Watch out for lead: Lead can harm the baby's developing brain and nervous system. If there is lead in your water supply (you can have it tested if you're not sure), you'll want to buy lead-free sterilized water or a special lead filter. Boiling it won't get the lead out. Also, don't boil water to be used to make formula in pots that contain lead. Pots made in the United States are supposed to be lead free.

Warming your baby's formula: If you want to warm your baby's formula, you can heat it by putting the bottle in a pan of water and warming it on the stove for a few minutes. Boiling or microwaving formula—or, for that matter, breast milk—can wreck some of the nutrients and vitamins it contains. Before you start feeding, squirt a few drops from the bottle onto the inside of your wrist to be sure it is warm, but not hot.

Feeding position: Formulas and bottles may be easier to give because even a semi-awake baby is likely to start sucking on a bottle nipple. But try to get the baby awake and responsive before you begin to feed with formula. Rock and sing to get the baby alert.

As we've said, careful positioning can make all the difference as a newborn baby first learns to feed. Even if your baby is squawking eagerly for food, take your time to get settled. Sit in a comfortable chair, preferably a rocking chair. Tilt him up to a 30 degree angle. Talk to him so he knows you are there. When he's really alert, and maybe even beginning to recognize the sensation of hunger, you can start the feeding. Hold him close. Be with him and enjoy it! Never feed a baby by leaving the bottle propped for him. Not only is it cold and impersonal, but he may choke and you wouldn't be there to rescue him.

As he suckles on the bottle, his face will soften, his hands will come up around the bottle, he will look up in your face as he works to suck down an ounce or two.

Bubbling and Burping

When he stops feeding, whether from breast or bottle, his face turns red and he begins to squirm. It may be time to bubble him. At first, you may need to put him up to your shoulder more often. Later, once or twice during a feeding should suffice.

A baby who gulps is gulping down air. A gulper needs more frequent bubbling. Put him up on your shoulder. Pat him or rub his back gently. Meanwhile, he'll look around, nuzzle into your shoulder, arch a bit so you know there's a bubble. He'll lay his head in the crook of your neck. All of a sudden, he'll arch backward to burp. Finally, it comes.

Nothing is as rewarding as a loud burping bubble. It's worth feeding a baby just to get a chance to burp him! If putting him up on your shoulder doesn't work, lay him quietly across your lap on his belly with his head turned sideways. Don't get frantic. Some babies don't have a bubble, particularly if they aren't noisy, gulping eaters. Breastfed babies are usually very effective eaters and may reward you with only one bubble at the end.

A little bit of spit-up is normal. If a lot of the feeding comes back, the baby may have a weak sphincter at the top of the stomach. (See *Spitting Up, Gastroesophageal Reflux, and Pyloric Stenosis* in Chapter Three.)

How Much to Feed
In each 24-hour period babies usually need 2½ to 3 ounces for every pound they weigh. At first, your newborn baby may drink only 2 or 3 ounces at each feeding. In the newborn period, a breastfed baby will nurse every 2 or 3 hours, or about 8 to 12 times a day. Although you'll want to work up to 10–15 minutes of nursing with each breast, your baby will take in most of your milk in the first 5–7 minutes. More time will help your breasts make more milk and satisfies your baby's need to suck.

A baby who is too quiet and doesn't wake at least every 4 hours should be awakened for feedings. Let your doctor know if your baby seems too sleepy to wake up for feedings on his own. Within 3 or 4 weeks, after the breast milk supply is steady, your baby will nurse less often but may be drinking 4 ounces at most feedings.

When to Feed

In the first weeks you will want to feed your baby on demand. He needs it, and if you are breastfeeding, on-demand feeding will also help to establish your milk supply. Eventually, though, you may feel so competent that you'll be able to push him toward a schedule. In fact, you may be ready for a schedule before your baby is. You're ready when you notice that you don't jump as quickly as you did at first when he starts to move or whimper. Schedules are made for parents and families. Babies will, with time, learn to fit into them.

Helping Your Baby Handle Hunger and Other Early Sensations

When a young baby is hungry, he of course needs to be fed. I never advise letting a baby "cry it out" when he's hungry. But as you and he get to know each other, you may feel confident enough to let your baby get a little fussy before you rush to feed him, so that he can become aware of this sensation himself. If you do, you'll need to wait and watch to see whether he can squirm around and find his own thumb or fingers to suck on. If he settles himself this way, you'll know the difference between fussing and hunger, and he'll have a chance to practice self-soothing—a skill that will serve him throughout life.

If you hold him, remember that he'll smell your breast milk (he'll know your smell from other women's smell by 3 to 5 days), and he may not quiet for you without a chance to nurse, even if he's not hungry. Let someone else play with him and see if he quiets for them.

Weight Gain and Your Baby's Growth

A newborn will lose weight in the first few days, as he waits for your milk and adjusts to the demands of his new world. He may not regain his birth weight until he is 8–10 days old. Then, he should gain about an ounce each day. He should weigh at least a pound more at the end of the first month. You

---

How to Know When Your Baby Is Hungry

1. In the first weeks, most of his crying is likely to be saying he is hungry. If he's been changed, does not soothe with gentle rocking and singing, and is not crying piercingly (a cry of pain), he's probably ready for a feeding.
2. If he's not been fed for an hour or more, it may be time to feed again. After a few weeks, he'll be able to take in more at each feeding and stretch out the time he can go before he's hungry again.
3. When a baby is ready to feed, he'll often lift and bob his head, open his mouth, and even smack his lips, and he'll try to suck on whatever comes his way.

needn't worry about how much milk your baby is getting as long as you feed him whenever he's hungry. You can tell your baby is adequately fed if he is urinating with each feeding, if his mouth is not dry, and if his eyes are not sunken. But your doctor should evaluate him right away if he's urinating less often or if such symptoms *are* present.

How to Know When Your Baby Has Had Enough

1. If you are bottle-feeding your baby, you'll be able to measure the amount he takes in at each feeding. Your baby should be waking up often enough for at least six feedings a day. If not, you'll need to rouse him.
2. If you are breastfeeding, you may need to go by other signs. To start with, your baby should soon be able to empty the first breast you offer, and often even the second.
3. A baby who settles contentedly after nursing has likely had enough.
4. A baby who frequently wets and soils diapers (at least six wet diapers each day, and for bottle-fed babies, at least a few soft, mushy, yellowish stools) is also probably a well-fed baby. Breastfed babies often go for a day or two between stools, and sometimes more, especially after the first few weeks.
5. Your baby's pediatrician will monitor your baby's growth by checking his weight, height, and head circumference. Although your baby may lose a little weight in the first week, he should catch up and make good progress thereafter.

Milk Allergies

A baby who cries a great deal or spits up a lot after each feeding should be examined by his pediatrician. He may have an allergy to the proteins in milk. This can cause stomach pains, fussiness, vomiting, and diarrhea. By 4 to 6 months, he may begin to develop a flat, peeling rash—eczema, which is another indication of milk protein sensitivity. Talk with your doctor about stopping the milk formula and changing to a substitute as soon as you recognize it. (There is an acne-like rash that all babies get at 4 to 6 weeks, which is not an allergic reaction but which may be confused with an allergic rash. It's simply a sign that the skin pores are beginning to function. Nothing to be done about that rash.) (See *Milk and Milk Allergies* in Chapter Three.)

Jaundice

Many babies have some jaundice after birth. Once outside the uterus, a new baby will need fewer red blood cells. The excess cells break up, releasing a substance called bilirubin that makes the skin appear yellow. The jaundice usually fades after a week or two. But if the bilirubin level gets too high or the excess remains for too long, it could damage the baby's brain. To prevent this from happening, special lights are used that actually help break down the bilirubin.

Breastfed babies are likely to get more jaundice, because the hormones in breast milk compete with the bilirubin to be broken down by the newborn baby's liver. But as far as we know, jaundice in a breastfed baby is usually not as serious and should subside eventually. Surprisingly, more frequent breastfeeding may help by stimulating the baby's digestive system to rid the body of bilirubin faster.

Premature babies are more likely to have jaundice earlier, and for longer. There are also a few unusual conditions (for example, incompatibility between the mother's and the baby's blood types) that can cause serious jaundice in the newborn period that require immediate attention and treatment. Blood type incompatibility should be screened for in routine prenatal visits. Once the baby is born, hospital staff should also check for jaundice and conditions that can cause it.

Watch for jaundice increasing in the first week or so. Watch the white of your baby's eyes and his skin for a yellow color. If his skin or the whites of his eyes look yellow, be sure to call your doctor.

Getting to Know One Another

As the first few weeks proceed, your baby will become easier and easier for you to care for. For one thing, you'll know him better. You will know his different cries (see our book *Calming Your Fussy Baby*), when he is crying to be fed, when you need to help him, and when he can first be given a chance to try to settle himself.

Both parents may find it fun to talk to him before a feeding—while the mother readies her breasts, or the father prepares a bottle of formula. It can be a lovely time for communication: "Hold on. You can do it. You can make it for just another minute until your milk is ready. Look at you—you did it. When we can talk together, you can wait!"

Parents will see that their baby knows the mother's voice (4 days), her smell (7 days), her face (10 days), and the father's voice and face (14 days). Each day, he is willing to wait a little longer for his feeding, as he becomes more and more fascinated with your faces and voices. He is learning to trust you, to know that when you speak to him or hold him, he can be sure you'll follow it up with a feeding.

Fussy Babies

Babies seem to know better than we do about when they need to be fed, and how much. It is usually safe to follow the baby's requests. Can you spoil a baby by picking him up or feeding him every time he cries? No, but try talking to him first. He may want to play or may be bored. Before rushing to feed him, find out what he's fussing about. For example, at the end of the day there is a fussy period of 1 to 3 hours from 3 to 12 weeks of age when hunger is not the issue (this kind of fussing is discussed in the next section).

Stretching Out Feedings

Parents' natural response to an agitated baby is to feed him. In the first weeks, when babies are growing so rapidly and need to be fed frequently, this is often what is needed. Most babies will quiet, and parents will feel successful. Feeding soon becomes the response to an upset baby. A new parent wonders, "How often can I feed him and not 'overfeed' him?" At first, it may be as often as every 1–2 hours—or twelve times a day and night for a week or so. By 4 to 6 weeks, he should be slowing down and stretching out feedings.

Over this period of time, the amount of breast milk or formula that a baby can take in at each feeding will slowly increase so that he can go for longer between feedings. Meanwhile, watch for the baby's own ways of calming himself when he is distressed but not really hungry.

He will learn to turn to his thumb or a pacifier, to bat at a toy hung safely over his crib by 12 weeks, a reachable toy by 16 weeks. These new ways of entertaining himself balance the gradual decrease in the frequency of the infant's feedings. Over time, a baby learns to recognize when he is hungry and to make it clear that it is time for a feeding. Then feedings can more precisely reward his growing awareness of his own hunger cycle. As he learns, he and his parents can begin to recognize that knowing when and how much he needs to feed is becoming his job.

3 Weeks

By 3 weeks, feedings should have become more predictable and enjoyable. Breastfeeding is now understood by all of you. But by 3 weeks, parents are often overwhelmed with exhaustion. Waking up every night for feeding is taking its toll, and the fatigue is building up. The awareness that the responsibility of being a parent is forever emerges now. With the fatigue, and with little evidence yet that the baby will ever get through a night without a feeding, forever seems like a very long time. To make this an even more challenging time, the end-of-the-day fussing can make a parent feel unrewarded. It can be comforting, though, for parents to realize how much they've already learned, how much they've already accomplished with the new routines they've set up.

Making Room for Fathers

The milk supplies of breastfeeding mothers should be reliable by 3 weeks. Introducing a bottle now won't interfere. Now a father can feed his baby too. He might start, for example, with a "night bottle" so that the mother can sleep a little longer. It can be a time when a father and his newborn are alone together and can get to know each other more intimately. He will discover how delicious it can be to hold his baby and look into his eyes, feeling his whole body sucking rhythmically, and then relaxing into sleep. Fathers can also help by fetching a sobbing baby from his crib to be breastfed, while a nursing mother settles into a comfortable position.

Although the father is helping, a mother is bound to feel jealous. She may not be aware of her competitive feelings, but find herself saying, "That's not the way you hold the baby. He's used to it this way." Or, "He likes to be burped every ounce. You give him too much at a time." I call this "gatekeeping." It will surface from time to time as a natural reaction to sharing a baby, a reaction that is to be expected.

Everyone who cares about the same baby will feel this competitive urge. Now is the time for each parent to try things out and find his or her own way. It's easy for one parent, often the mother, to feel superior right after she's been through an anxious learning period of her own. But each parent needs to go through their own trials and errors and learn. It will help to discuss your feelings with each other. When something goes even slightly wrong, everyone becomes upset. Being able to blame someone else is a relief: "If you did it *my* way, that would never have happened." But remember that everyone else is vulnerable too. The other parent, or a close relative, may even withdraw from helping you, or from getting to know your baby better. However, when parents can support each other, a baby will benefit from a special relationship with each parent.

Checkup for Babies
Your baby's doctor or nurse practitioner should check him by 2 or 3 weeks of age for progress with feeding and growth, for dehydration, jaundice, and withdrawal from any medication or drugs taken during pregnancy. At the same time, she or he should check the mother for postpartum depression.

Getting Ready for a Schedule
As the baby begins to establish his own rhythms for waking and sleep states, he will begin to be more predictable. I recommend demand feeding (feeding your baby whenever he's hungry) in the first weeks so you can get to know him, and he can get to know you. As you push him to wait 3 hours between feedings, you are already letting him learn to wait until he feels hungry. This rhythm will help him mature in his feeding and sleep cycles. He is getting ready for a schedule that will fit with the rest of the family's. This will make life so much easier for everyone.

Irritable, End-of-the-Day Fussing

After the first few weeks and just when life seems to be settling down, the fussiness that often starts at 3 weeks can come as a shock to new parents. At 3 weeks, a baby is likely to start fussing more regularly at the end of the day, almost demanding to be picked up, to be held, to be rocked, to be fed. He may fuss inconsolably for 1 to 3 hours every day. Parents often try everything possible to calm this fussing: putting his bassinet on the washing machine, using a loud radio or TV, carrying him or feeding him almost constantly. A baby may even stop during all of this, and retreat into a light sleep to shut out all the commotion. But as soon as the distraction stops, he's likely to start up again. In fact, he may fuss longer as a result of all of these desperate, but vain efforts.

This has been called "colic" or "irritable end-of-the-day crying." We describe it in our book *Calming Your Fussy Baby: The Brazelton Way.* I like to think of this fussing as a baby's response to an overload of stimulation. It is as if the baby needed to let off steam at the end of each demanding new day. After the fussy period, you may eventually notice that he begins to eat and sleep better for the next 24 hours. In other words, this fussing may be serving a purpose—letting off steam after each overloaded day. By 3 months, when he's learned to do other things—smiling, gurgling, watching his world—he is likely to stop his fussy periods and to substitute alert times instead.

What to do? Try everything that might soothe him. Check him all over to be sure he isn't sick or that something isn't causing pain. (A cry of pain, though, is usually different—a piercing, more insistent cry.) If he's okay but nothing works, resign yourself. Let him work it out for 10–15 minutes at a time. Then pick him up to cuddle and soothe him. Let him suckle on warm water and bubble him. If he's desperate, you may even want to feed him more often. But you'll quickly recognize that he's not really hungry. Put him down several times to work it out. After it's over, cuddle him to let him know how glad you are and how you wish you could have helped more.

Spitting Up

This may be the time when spitting up after feedings may be getting worse. If propping your baby at a 30 degree angle, burping, and gentle handling don't work, let your pediatrician know. She or he will check for dehydration and make sure that your baby's weight is adequate. Breast milk is less likely than cow's milk to be regurgitated. However, if your baby is not simply spitting up, but instead vomiting violently, so that stomach contents seem to shoot straight out of his mouth a foot or more, have your doctor evaluate him right away. There are many different possible causes. Many can be readily remedied but need urgent attention. An uncommon one is pyloric stenosis. (See *Spitting Up, Gastroesophageal Reflux, and Pyloric Stenosis* in Chapter Three.)

Bowel Movements

Bowel movements have been through several changes. From the black sticky goo of meconium to softer, greenish stools, and finally cocoa-colored stools. Breastfed babies' stools don't smell bad, but formula-fed babies' stools do. Don't worry about frequent stools if your baby is feeding and growing well. At least one a day is likely with formula, even up to five or six. After about 3 weeks on breast milk, a baby may have stools less often—only one every few days or even only one a week. The wait may frighten you at first, but when it comes you'll know it's okay by its mushy, soupy consistency.

2 Months

As a balance to the fussing at the end of the day that may be peaking now, a baby has learned many new ways to win over his parents. By the age of 2 months, a baby has learned to smile and to coo. These are tremendous assets. Few parents or caregivers can resist. As a smile is coming on, he will wriggle with his whole body. His legs flex, his arms wave gently above his head, his whole face brightens, his forehead wrinkles, his cheeks rise, his color increases, and last of all, a *smile*! With it a gurgle, then a "goo." By this time, a parent is in ecstasy, responding with all sorts of playful rituals, blowing bubbles on his stomach, tickling his cheeks. Anything to produce another smile or a gurgle.

Other new skills may go unnoticed. For example, as a bottle begins to be readied, he may quiet to listen. As the nipple appears, his face becomes even more serious. His limbs become completely still—or more active. His mouth opens in anticipation. A breastfed baby may start rooting with his face and mouth toward the side where his mother's body is. He may already refuse a bottle or any substitute for his mother's smell and his mother's breast when she is near.

He knows already where his milk is coming from, and he prepares for it. His body arches around his mother, his arms and hand go up to contain his mother's breast. His mouth opens as the breast is bared. He will be demonstrating his stored memories—of the many, many feedings he will have experienced by now. His memories have formed an "expectancy"—early evidence of memory storage and a healthily developing brain.

Mothers, Fathers, and Strangers

An even more exciting observation can be made by now. He can differentiate between his mother, his father, and other adults. His fingers, his toes, his mouth, his legs—his whole body will behave differently for each of these adults. He has already learned what to expect from each one of them. This learning is built on repeated experiences. Every time his mother looms in sight, for example, he knows how she will behave.

In our filmed experiments, we place a 2-month-old infant in a reclining baby chair. When his mother is asked to "go in and play with him," she will always do the same thing. She will quietly sit down in front of the baby chair. She'll form an envelope around the infant with her voice, her face, and hands. Her hands will gently embrace her baby's buttocks, holding his legs to keep them from jerking. She'll softly coo to him. The baby will coo back, and his mother will dimple with joy. She'll coo again, jiggling her infant's buttocks to keep him engaged. This will be repeated three or four times until the baby tires of it.

Meanwhile, the 2-month-old's arms, his fingers, his toes are reaching out, then curling slowly back again, smoothly moving in an arc toward the mother, then curling back again. His face softens, then brightens. All of this occurs in smooth, cycling movements toward, then withdrawing from, his mother. This is predictable behavior and will say to the mother, "I know you and what to expect of you!"

Since fathers never behave like mothers, we can tell by the movement of any part of the baby's body when his father has come into view, or called to him from across the room. As he comes in to play with his baby in the baby chair, everything about the baby goes up. Eyes, eyebrows, cheeks, mouth, hands, fingers, toes, legs—all react with him in a jerky gesture, as if expecting to play. We call the baby's look a "pounce-face." It certainly says, "Play with me." And his father will. He pokes the baby from toes to head, over and over. Meanwhile the baby chortles, jerks his extremities and his face lights up; this reaction to his father is predictable and says, "I know what you'll do!"

With these expectations for excitement, how could he care about food? A father who is serious about feeding his baby had better play with him first. When the infant begins to tire, to lose enthusiasm, to turn his head away to avoid his father's gaze, then, and only then, can the father cuddle him, rock him gently, croon to him, and, finally, offer him a bottle. Even a determined breastfed baby may be ready to accept it.

New Gains, New Routines

The baby has gained about 2 more pounds since the 3-week checkup. His feedings are more predictable now. He may even begin to stretch out his periods of sleep at night. He may have learned to wait—briefly—before you can get to him to soothe his hungry cries. On your way to him, stop out of sight, and call to see whether he can accept you on faith yet.

His feedings should be about 5–6 ounces at a time now. On the breast, this amount comes in the first 5–10 minutes, but the sucking on each breast soothes him, and is often pleasurable for mothers too.

Colic

At 2 months, many babies are at the peak of their end-of-the-day fussiness. Many parents find that their babies can soothe themselves—at least briefly—by sucking on a pacifier or, better still, by nursing. Prolonged nursing will not overfeed a baby.

Bowel Movements

Bowel movements stay the same as they were. One or two a day on a formula—mushy, yellow to brown. He may squirm and turn red as he produces them, but he'll relax once he's done. If you see any blood, be sure to report this to your doctor. Small streaks of red blood may appear in a baby's stools when a hardened stool makes a small crack in the baby's anus. When this happens, try to soften his bowel movements by giving him an ounce of prune juice and 2 ounces of water to drink. To help heal any crack in the surface of the anus, rub a little petroleum jelly around the area with the tip of your little finger.

Breastfed babies' bowel movements are unpredictable. They can occur from ten times a day to one every tenth day. As long as they are soft and mushy and don't hurt the baby, you needn't worry. Rarely, a stool may have a bit of digested brown blood from a mother's cracked nipple. This will warn you that you had better take care of your nipple by applying a lanolin ointment. You may need to ask your doctor about avoiding feeding on that side until the crack heels.

Feedings at this age should be fun, and you and the infant should look forward to them—for play as much as for food.

Solid Foods?

Milk is the most important food for your baby in the first year. A baby's swallowing reflexes are not well coordinated enough to handle solids until at least 4 to 5 months of age. Solids fed to babies earlier are likely to come through their guts undigested. Their undeveloped guts can be stressed by giving solids too soon. There is also evidence that feeding certain solid foods to babies this young might cause later allergies.

4 Months

Feedings should be more predictable now. Nearly all babies will have settled into a rhythm of 3–4 hours between feedings. Each feeding now is more likely to last for a predictable amount of time. A bottle feeding may take 10 to 15 minutes plus bubbling time. A breastfeeding can last 20 minutes, and sometimes more—with burping and bubbling. Quiet talking and gentle play, so rewarding, may add a little more time. The baby takes in half of his feeding in the first 2 minutes, and 80–90 percent in the first 4 minutes. If he falls asleep after that, he's probably had enough. But if he wants to nurse for longer, and if his mother wants him to, this can be a delicious time for closeness. The baby certainly won't be overfed with these longer feedings.

It has always seemed to me that a parent who takes a few minutes in the beginning to talk and hug and alert the baby, to calm him down if he's frantic, will have a more rewarding, smoother feed.

You probably know your baby's cries by now. The intense, end-of-the-day fussing should be over by now. An alert period of smiling and interacting may have replaced it. By now parents will feel more confident about knowing their baby and what to expect with each cry. Hunger cries are like no others, and you and your baby both know them.

A number of questions will linger in parents' minds during this period:

Q: Will I spoil him if I feed him every time he cries?

A: I don't believe that a baby this young can be spoiled. But be sure you recognize his ways of telling you about his other needs. He will tell you several different things by his cries. Not all cries are hunger cries. There are different reasons for them, such as boredom and the need to play, or fatigue, and the need to be put down to sleep. Each of these needs, and others, are expressed with different cries. Look for them, and you will feel more in touch with him.

Q: He seems to want to eat so often. What can I do to hold him off?

A: This is the age when you can begin to respect your baby's newly developing abilities. When you go to him in less than 3 hours, try to substitute play for your feeding for awhile. He is probably ready for some play on his own.

Hang a few colored objects (e.g., plastic spoons) over his crib, so he can look at them as they twinkle in the light. These should be removed when the baby can successfully reach, and they should be fastened securely enough that he or an older sibling can't pull them down. Prop him at a 30 degree angle so he can look at them and listen to them. You may be surprised to see that, with the chance to watch, listen, and try to reach, he'll become intrigued.

He will discover that he can play by himself, handling his boredom and enjoying his waking time between feedings. This certainly will help you—and think what it may mean to him to sense that he can take care of some of his own needs. Then you can both gratefully enjoy the reward of a feeding at the 4-hour mark. You have both worked for it!

Q: Why does he wake up to feed every 4 hours at night?

A: The 4-hour sleep cycle at night is a normal one. Actually, you may be lucky. At least your child sleeps for 4-hour stretches at night instead of waking more often or staying awake at night and sleeping during the day. But this is a good time to begin to push him to learn how to sleep longer at night. As his brain begins to mature, he may be ready to go longer at night.

Continuing to pick up and feed him every few hours could lead to sleep troubles. Feedings every 4 hours at night may not be the answer now. Learning to get himself to sleep may be.

I have found that when a baby has begun to learn how to get himself back down, interrupting the 4-hour cycle can help break it. Wake him at 10:00 or 11:00 P.M. before he wakes himself. Feed him an extra feeding then, without play or exciting interactions. Put him down before he's asleep, leaving him to get himself back down to sleep. The extra feeding can break the every-four-hour cycle, and it may help him learn to get himself to sleep and to sleep longer at night. It has worked to push many of my patients toward an 8-hour sleep at night. Feedings may help, but they won't contribute to the real job of "learning how to sleep." (See our book *Sleep: The Brazelton Way.*)

Solids

Some parents feel that solids will help prolong a 4-month-old's sleep. If you do, be sure you start with a single-grain cereal, preferably one that does not contain wheat. Many pediatricians recommend a rice-based cereal to start with. Avoid using a mixture, because your baby might well be allergic to one of the grains, but you won't know which one.

Some solid foods can cause allergies, so be careful when you start each new one. Wait at least a week after introducing each new one to see whether your baby develops signs of an allergy. Either a rash that often starts on the face or an upset stomach can warn you to stop giving him the new food. Eczema—dry, flaky skin—or other signs can appear if a baby is allergic.

Prepared baby cereals should be fortified with iron, since many babies begin to need extra iron by 4 to 6 months of age. Until then, babies draw on the iron supplies they received from their mothers before they were born.

Your baby will have a greater risk of developing food allergies if food allergies and eczema run in the family. If this is the case, wait until your infant is 6 months old before starting solids. If you do feel that you should restrict your baby's diet because of a family history of food allergies, be sure to ask your pediatrician to help you make sure your baby's nutritional needs are still being met. She or he may also refer you to a registered dietitian (see *Allergies to Foods* and *Nutritional Needs* in Chapter Three.)

When you first start solids, before the evening feeding, you can expect a few new challenges and questions:

1. The baby will have to learn how to swallow. He has been sucking his feeding down so far. Learning to swallow involves using muscles of the back of the tongue and throat. He may gag on solids the first few times—and even choke. Slow up, and give him time to learn. A bit of very liquid cereal on a tiny spoon can be a start. Let him suck

it off. If he's ready for solids, in three or four days, he'll be an expert. Some infants take a little longer to develop this kind of coordination of the tongue and throat muscles. And some may have a very sensitive gag reflex, gagging and choking whenever solid food touches the back of their throats. These infants may need at least another month before they are ready for solids.

2. How much solid food should you give? One or two table-spoons mixed with formula or breast milk is adequate for the next few months.

3. Will he like it? Probably not, at first. A baby makes a face at any new food. He'll roll it around in his mouth, spit it back slowly. You'll have to be patient, and keep offering it until he tires. It also helps to keep offering him the new food again at each feeding. Many babies and young children need to get used to a new taste or texture before they're ready to swallow it. After five to fifteen introductions to the new food, it will no longer be new. They will eventually accept a new food when it is repeatedly offered in this way. But don't force it—ever. Just offer your baby a spoonful a few times. When he resists, respect his signals, and try again at the next meal. You don't want him to connect new tastes or textures with struggles. Then he'll be more likely to refuse them—for good.

4. At 4 months, a baby may try to grab for the spoon. When he succeeds, let him keep it to hold and play with. While he's doing this, you can use another one. If he goes for

that one, you may need to let him keep one for each hand. Use a third spoon to keep on feeding him!

5. Can solids be started later? Yes, indeed. Not all babies are ready at 4 months. I'd wait until he seemed hungry at night. Don't wait too long, though. Most babies need a chance to begin to try out new and different textures by about 6 months of age if they are to learn to handle these foods in their mouths.

6. What to do if a baby won't nurse or drink formula after solids? Reverse the order. Milk is still most important, so give it first. Solids can follow, since they don't matter as much at this age.

7. If a baby begins to get a dry scaly rash on his face, should solids be stopped? Not all solids. If you've been waiting at least a week before introducing each new solid, just eliminate the most recent one. Then don't try that food again. With his diet as restricted as it is at this age, you have a chance to check each food for its allergic potential for your baby. It is a real advantage to find out which ones will work and which ones won't.

8. After 2 weeks of cereal at the evening feeding, you may be ready to introduce other solids. Prop your baby up in a baby chair or on a pillow to feed him solids. Expect him to push them out with his tongue. One to two tablespoons at each meal is enough. While you feed him facing him, he will play with you as he eats. He'll reach for your face. He'll kick out with his legs and rub his feet together.

Expect him to flip his head from side to side when he's bored or when he's finished with solids.

How to Avoid Allergies While Introducing Solid Foods

1. Start one new solid food at a time. This gives you a chance to test the baby's sensitivity to it. If you can ferret out which solids he can't tolerate, you may be able to protect your baby from eczema and other allergic reactions to foods.
2. Continue with that food for a week.
3. Read the labels on baby food jars and cans. If there is more than one kind of food in a container, this is not the time to introduce it.
4. Don't use mixtures, because they can be loaded with different kinds of cereals to which you don't want to expose the baby.
5. Don't start solids until your baby is at least 4 months old.

New Interests, and No Interest in Feeding

A new "touchpoint" in feeding is coming. Somewhere between 4 and 5 months, a baby just won't stay at the breast or bottle. He will jerk away to pay attention to every new sight or sound. Unless you feed him in a dark, quiet room, it's almost impossible to keep him eating. This is because at this age there is a new burst in awareness of sights and sounds. He has "suddenly" become aware of how exciting his world can be. He wants to observe, listen, and take in every new cue that he can. Along with this, his eyes now can focus on more distant objects, allowing him to take in not just your face, but the toys on the floor at the other end of the room! Eating seems so much less important right now.

What to do? Be patient. Be aware of the reason for this new burst in development. Since he is distracted by the excitement of the world around him, try feeding him in a calm, quiet, darkened room. Don't expect him to drink for more than a few minutes before he will want to stop and look around. He'll get enough in four feedings during the day. On the breast, he'll drink 3–4 ounces in the first 5 minutes. This challenging period will last a week. You may feel rejected or as if something has gone wrong. This is often attributed to "teething." Teething may be playing a role, but it's much more likely to be this burst in learning. Enjoy it!

Teething

Teething can indeed make feedings more difficult. Everything is blamed on teething in a baby over 4 months of age. Every refusal of food is blamed on teething. That may be the reason, if you can see swollen gums in the front of the lower jaw. A new tooth acts like a splinter—a foreign body that makes gums swell. When a baby sucks, more blood rushes in to the already engorged gums, and they hurt.

If he sucks on his fingers a lot, if he fusses when he first latches on to the nipple, he is likely to be teething. Teething may cause a baby to rub on his ears as if they hurt. One can confuse this rubbing and fussing for an earache. The reason is that the nerves to the teeth go through the ear area, and it is comforting to rub on the surrounding area.

If you want to help, wash your finger and rub his lower front jaw—inside his mouth, just above where his lip meets his gum—to reduce the swelling. He'll hate it at first, then he'll settle down to enjoy it. You can manage his teething pain this way. You'll notice that he looks forward to your finger, and rubs his own gums as he sucks on his own fingers.

The age at which a baby starts teething usually runs in families. My children didn't get their first tooth until late in the first year. I worried all along. "When is her tooth coming? Will she ever get teeth?" I needn't have worried. My mother said, "Berry, you didn't get a tooth until you were a year old. Then they all came at once. But they were better for the wait."

Grandparents and Other Caregivers

At 4 months, the earliest signs of stranger awareness emerge. The baby will already have learned differences between parents and what to expect from them. He will have stored this information and be ready to behave differently with each parent—and with others. Although this new ability is just beginning to take hold, grandparents can already expect to be looked over carefully before the baby relaxes to interact with them. Caregivers or baby-sitters may also need to respect a baby's awareness of the different people in his life when they attempt to feed him.

I would suggest to grandparents or caregivers who want to feed the baby that they get to know him first. Play with him quietly without looking him in the eye. Pick him up quietly, and gently. Even then, don't look him in the face. Don't try to jazz him up. Don't try to make him laugh or coo at you. Just sit and rock him. Fit into his rhythms. As he relaxes for you, you can feel his body become less tense. Then, and only then, you can sing and talk gently to him. As he begins to root around, looking for a feeding, then you can offer him a bottle. If he begins to suck, you can be grateful. Keep still, and don't overload him. When he falls into the burst-pause pattern we described earlier, use the pauses to communicate gently with him. Look down quietly at him when he pauses. Sing a quiet song. Jiggle him gently to keep him awake to communicate with you and to finish his feeding.

But remember that he's aware of you as a stranger and is likely to be wary of all the differences from his usual source of food—your smells, your voice, your arms, your rhythms. The burst-pause pattern is a time for learning—in this case, learning about you as a stranger—but your behavior is likely to be painfully reminiscent of all the usual cues that he associates with his parents. His willingness to accept you at all right now is a major accomplishment.

6 Months

Feedings now can be exciting—or disappointing. It depends on how you take them. The 4- or 5-month-old's refusal of the breast or bottle in order to look around usually lasts only briefly. But the baby is now alerted to his exciting environment as well as his ability to engage in it. He knows by now that if he stops sucking to look up at you, he can coo or gurgle to capture your attention. He can interrupt feedings to make them last longer and longer.

Solid Foods

Some babies begin to turn to solids now and away from milk feedings. If so, begin with milk first, and offer solids afterward. Milk is more important to a rapidly growing baby than solids are, although by 6 months, babies may need more iron. Iron-fortified cereal is one source. Pureed meat is another. Ask your pediatrician to help you be sure your baby is getting enough iron at this critical stage.

Always prop the baby at a 30 or 40 degree angle for solids. Lower than that, and he might choke and swallow them down "the wrong way." Higher than that, and he will keep flopping over, instead of eating. You will want to try to ensure that his first experience with new tastes and food textures is not a frightening one.

Avoiding Food Allergies

Hopefully none of the new foods you have introduced so far have caused rashes or stomach upsets. It is still wise to introduce only one new food at a time, so that you can identify the specific food responsible for any allergic reaction. Sometimes I have seen the addition of new solids seem to uncork a mild cow's milk allergy. The milk and solids may act like building blocks that pile up to make a tower. In some babies, milk alone might not set off an allergic skin reaction like eczema. But add on more mildly allergenic solids, and the tower falls—a skin rash appears.

This is another time for you to be sure of each food your baby is exposed to and to watch to see which ones have caused an allergic reaction, before his environment and his diet become more complicated. Ask your baby's doctor or nurse for a list of foods most likely to cause allergies (common foods that cause allergic reactions include cow's milk, soy protein products, eggs—especially egg whites—peanuts, shellfish, and occasionally gluten—found in foods made from wheat, rye, oats, and barley), especially if you have family reasons to anticipate allergies. If an allergic reaction (such as a skin rash or diarrhea) develops, discontinue the offending food. Don't assume, though, that a single bout of diarrhea or a rash is a sign of food allergy, as there are also other causes for them. Ask your pediatrician to help you be sure that the baby's symptoms are really due to an allergy. (See *Allergies* and *Milk and Milk Allergies* in Chapter Three.)

Solids and Breastfeeding

If a mother who is breastfeeding is away during the day, she may need to take an extra step to keep up milk production now that her baby is eating other foods too. In order to keep her breasts stimulated, a working mother should try feeding her baby twice in the evening—once when she gets home, and again before going to bed. This, plus the morning feeding, and pumping once or twice at work, should certainly keep her milk coming.

Solids and Sleep

The addition of solids may not have helped the baby to mature in his sleep-wake cycles. Others may have told you that he'll "sleep through" when you give him cereal at night. But the job of helping him "learn" to sleep through is not just a matter of having a full stomach (see our book *Sleep: The Brazelton Way*). Don't be discouraged.

The spurt of interest in sights and sounds that disrupted his sleep pattern and feeding at 4 months should have passed by now. But he may still need to be taught to get himself back down to sleep after each 4-hour waking. If you are still feeding him every 4 hours, you are setting yourself up as part of his sleep-wake pattern. You may have to reconsider this approach as you head for bed yourself.

As we suggested earlier, you may want to try waking him at 10:00 or 11:00 P.M. to break his 4-hour cycle of waking. Rock him, sing quietly to him, feed him, and get him into a sleepy state—but don't put him down asleep. He won't learn anything that way about getting himself to sleep. Put him down when he's quiet but still awake. Then encourage him to put himself to sleep: "You can do it. You can do it yourself." You may need to rub his back, or sit nearby, but don't hold him, unless you want to remain a necessary part of his sleep-wake cycles.

If your baby can find his thumb or a pacifier, if he can squirm himself into a comfortable position, he'll have learned to become independent at night. He can rouse and get himself down the next time he wakes up—at 2:00 A.M.—without feeding.

Sitting Up—A New Skill, a New Position for Feeding

As your baby is learning to sit, he may be able to adjust gradually to a high chair. Prop him at an upright angle that he likes. But as you strap him, be sure he's not too upright. He'll sag and need to use one or both arms to support himself, like a tripod, when he tries to sit. He'll need to use both arms to hold himself for long in any upright position. He'll get frustrated and tired easily, so be sure he is able to flop back into a more comfortable position. He'll need it for the feeding and reaching tussle that you both will be facing.

Reaching—A New Skill, a New Challenge for Feeding

The newest threat to feeding is the baby's latest skill—reaching. At first, leaning back, he will have learned to reach with both arms at once. But by 6 months, he can prop his sagging body with one arm while he reaches out for your spoon with the other. As you bring in a loaded spoonful of cereal mush, he'll suddenly reach for it and turn it over to spill. Give him a spoon of his own—to bang with, to mouth, to fill up his hand just as you offer him a new taste.

Have fun with his new reach. Try something new! Offer him a spoon with its handle horizontal at first, and then turn it vertically. Watch to see whether he's ready yet to anticipate this change as he reaches out to grasp it. Soon, he may begin to turn his hand while it is still several inches away from the spoon to shape his grasp and anticipate the position of the spoon. He will be demonstrating his new capacity to respond to new visual information by changing his plan about how he will use his body. He may even look up at you to twinkle as he recognizes your new game.

Reaching for Food, Reaching for You

Enjoy his new ability to reach for you. Let him reach for your face and your mouth. As he explores your mouth, he'll be making connections between your mouth and his. If you smack your lips, he may smack his. If you sputter, he may sputter too. So be careful. Imitation is coming fast, and he'll learn new tricks to add to reaching for the spoon, all to divert your feeding efforts in the next few months. You'll enjoy them if you see them as his early steps—in getting ready to take control and feed himself on his own!

Feeding—A Time for Intimacy

Feeding is a wonderful time for learning about each other. First words—"Dada" for play, "Mama" for help when there's trouble—may even surface at feeding times. Meals will become more complicated as your baby works—little by little—toward self-feeding. You will be wise to think up new ways to let him become more and more independent. Be ready for him to shut his mouth when he's tired of a solid food, or to turn his head away; and be ready—in a flash—to reach out your hand to catch the spray of chewed-up carrots or peas he suddenly decides to offer you!

A Daily Schedule

For healthy 6-month-olds, I usually recommend a daily schedule that can eventually look like the following example. Exact amounts vary with factors such as a baby's size and activity level.

7:00 A.M.	Milk feeding
8:30 A.M.	Fruit, cooked and strained
11:00 A.M.	Diluted fruit juice or water. No more than 3–4 ounces of juice per day. No fruit drinks and no juice at all before 6 months of age. Try serving juice only in a sippie cup so that your baby never gets used to juice in his bottle. Don't let juice take the place of milk and important solid foods. (While limiting juice, there's no need to hold back on water.)
Noon	Cooked and strained meat and vegetable, milk feeding
3:00 P.M.	Water or juice, and perhaps a solid food snack
5:00 P.M.	Cereal and fruit (cooked and strained)
6:30 P.M.	Milk again
9:30–10:00 P.M.	Fourth milk feeding, if necessary

This schedule is a goal, not easily reached with babies who want to be fed more often. If you are breastfeeding, don't rush to eliminate feedings. You want to keep your breasts stimulated often enough to keep the milk coming. When you are feeding solids, watch him reach for your breast or for the bottle. He knows this is still the most important food you give him.

8 Months

The Reassurance of Routines and Regular Times for Feeding

By now, feeding times are set. Most babies are used to the three-meals-a-day routine and regular snack times. Snacks in the morning before a nap and in the afternoon after a nap are needed, since 8-month-olds' stomachs are small and hold less at each feeding than those of older children. Also, 8-month-olds are more active and need more food for energy. Babies this age are beginning to have a clearer idea of when they are hungry. Solids and milk feedings are likely to be given together now for everybody's convenience. When the baby begins to fall apart in the late afternoon, everyone knows "He's hungry. We'd better drop everything and feed him." They're right!

New Social Skills

He knows now how to demand attention and get it. At 8 months, he can look at his parents' faces to know their intent. "Are they going to get my food?" or "Are they getting themselves ready to sit down and feed me?" If he's not reassured by the silent answer to his questions that he is now able to read from their faces, he can let out such disturbing cries that no one can resist. This ability to read the faces of those who are known and important to him is a new achievement. It allows for a new kind of sociability at mealtimes. Now that the baby is beginning to feed himself, this new social skill will help him find new ways of feeling close to family members at mealtimes. Ultimately, this sociability is one of the most important motivations for healthy eating.

Stranger Anxiety

This new ability, however, is also accompanied by a new kind of recognition called "stranger anxiety," which can affect his tolerance of those other than his parents who try to feed him. The 8-month-old will be able to compare his mother's and his aunt's ability to read his cues—and find differences that leave him more comfortable with his mother.

Don't plan for anyone else to be very successful in feeding the baby right now. If someone else must feed him, warn the new person not to look him in the face and to quietly distract him by presenting an interesting toy first. Then, fill his hands with two objects, so he can't grab the spoon. Hold the spoon up—filled with his favorite solid food. Expect him to resist a new or substitute person for a week or so.

New Skills, New Dangers—Creeping, Grasping

Creeping or squirming along the floor is another new skill. With it comes the hunger to use another new skill—grasping—to capture and gather up fuzz, bits of dirt, anything left on the floor. An 8-month-old will always bring them to his mouth to explore and even swallow them. Parents will find it necessary to search the floor for small objects and to sweep more often than ever (as if there wasn't already too much to do!) before letting the baby creep around. I always suggest that parents get down on their hands and knees and creep around themselves to see what dangers lurk in the newly mobile child's expanding world. This grasping ability is also useful for self-feeding.

A New Discovery—Fingers!

In the first month or so after a baby first begins to sit, he needs his hands to prop himself up and to keep from falling from his sitting position. Up until recently, his hands were busy, forming a secure tripod. But once a baby learns to sit and balance reliably, his arms and hands are free for other activities. The next step is the fine-tuning of hand and finger movements. His fingers are such fascinating instruments for him. He can watch them. He can guide them. He can use them to ferret out small objects. Of course the 8-month-old will insist on using his fingers in a task as exciting and important as feeding.

The Beginning of Self-Feeding

Once fingers have become available to him in this way, the 8-month-old's hands become an extension of his mouth in exploring his universe. He is still a long way from replacing his mouth with his fingers to examine his world, but he's getting started. As he picks up bits of food or objects to take to his mouth, watch for this transition. He'll begin to touch a Cheerio, as if to ask, "Why haven't I noticed the hole in it before? How fascinating!" He'll take a Cheerio in his hand, try to poke a finger into the hole. When it sticks to his sticky finger and he can lift it without a grasp, he'll look up triumphantly, as if to say, "Look what I can do now!"

Pointing

The 8-month-old is learning to refine his hand grasp. Whereas he has probably been content to scrape up mush or a solid object with his whole hand, he is now beginning to separate his fingers. As he does, he learns he can point. He can point to an object and grunt—to get it! Pointing is a powerful new way to communicate. Now, simply by extending his index finger he can say—"look at that!" or "I want that" or even express hunger or a food preference, when he points to his bottle, or to the food on your plate. Pointing is also a social accomplishment. Your baby can now seem to say, with his pointing finger: "Let's look at that together." A forefinger also becomes a new way to explore not just food, but light sockets, so watch out! Protective socket caps are a must! A baby this age will need to poke at everything you offer him to eat. His hands will get messy. Let them.

Pincer Grasp

Most exciting of all, the 8-month-old learns that he can use his forefinger and his thumb to pick up objects. Sometime in the next month or so he will discover that he can trap even a small bit of food—a baby biscuit, or a tiny piece of meat—between his thumb and index finger. This is a momentous new triumph for him. He has learned the "pincer grasp." Of course he is ex-

cited. This means he can also more easily pick up small dangerous objects—for example, thumb tacks, chips of lead paint,
coins—to put in his mouth. So the caution about everything
within his reach that we mentioned earlier becomes even more
important.

New Skills for Feeding

When a child is working on all these new abilities, it may be a
touchpoint. These emerging skills may result in a temporary
backsliding of other ones, in other areas of development. This
is a time for parents to understand the backward steps and to
see them as a kind of preparation for the new developmental
advances ahead. Finger feeding is a major step toward independence and toward making choices of foods. These choices
need to be understood from his perspective: his excitement at
these new powers will become a major motivation to learn to
feed himself on his own.

In addition, a baby this age can now become interested in
how a cup and a spoon work. He may take one while you are
feeding him from another. He'll bang it on his tray or table.
He'll poke it in the mush you feed him. He'll take the cup to
hold it by the rim, then by its handle. If you are daring enough
to put anything in it to see if he'll feed himself, he'll turn it up-
side down. Use a little water in it if you want. Another solution,
of course, is a sippie cup, which has a firmly attached cover.
And don't put the food bowl on his table, or you can expect to
see it on top of his head!

With his new pincer grasp, your baby is now able to hold a piece of food, and he wants to use this new skill! In order to keep him interested in feedings now, it is wise to start with one or two soft bits of food, such as a small piece of banana. Put them on his high chair tray before you start to try to spoon him his solid purees. As he works to pick them up with his thumb and index finger, you can spoon-feed him.

Finger Foods

When you first put down two bits of food on his high chair tray, he'll drop them over the side. Ignore this, and offer two more. You might want to put down a tarpaulin under his high chair. Or let the dog clean up. Otherwise, you can expect your floor to be dotted with dropped scraps of food.

The bits of food need to have special appeal, especially at first. They need to be firm enough to pick up and soft enough to swallow whole, or to soften before swallowing. Bits of cereal foods work nicely. Cheerios are perfect because they dissolve quickly into a mush the baby can swallow. Other good choices are bits of soft fruit, soft bits of cooked hamburger (not too dry), cooked vegetables or macaroni, tofu, soft cheese, and bits of the soft part of toast. All of these will soften and be easy to swallow.

How to Handle Choking

Be ready to help your baby with choking and swallowing dangerous small objects off the floor. You should have a guide to infant CPR (such as that provided in the *Children's Hospital*

Guide to Your Child's Health and Development—see Bibliography) handy. Read it before you start feeding solid foods. You can also take a CPR course from the Red Cross or a local hospital, or sometimes through an employer or health club.

If the baby is able to cry or cough on his own, let him cough up the offending piece of food or object. But if he can't give a good cough and is having trouble breathing, but is conscious, put him belly down on your forearm, head down, supporting his head and neck firmly with your hand. With a heavy baby you many need to support that arm with your knees. With the heel of your other hand, whack him four or five times between the shoulder blades. If this doesn't help him cough up whatever is stuck, put your free hand and arm over his back, and turn him over onto his back, supporting his head and neck, keeping his head below his body. Then use two or three fingers to press—up to five times—on the infant's chest, on his breastbone. Make sure your fingers are just below the level of his nipples, but not at the very bottom of his breastbone. Keep alternating these chest thrusts and back blows until the child coughs up the piece of food or small object.

If your infant appears to be unconscious or not breathing, try to rouse him by touching his shoulder, and shout for someone to call 911 for emergency help so that you can stay with your baby. If no one is nearby, call 911 yourself, but keep your baby with you. In either case, then start infant CPR. The Heimlich maneuver is not recommended for babies under 1 year. All parents with a baby under 8 months will want to have instructions handy on maneuvers to help a choking baby. Put a sticker with emergency numbers on your phones. (See also *Choking* in Chapter Three.)

New Skills, New Safety Concerns

Prevention is the best remedy. Again, explore your floors and close your cabinets. Don't leave small, easily swallowed objects on the floor or in the baby's reach. Feed him only two small bits at a time. Be ready with water or juice or even milk to help him wash the bits down. Meanwhile, don't hover over him to put pressure on him to eat. A baby this age may respond to your pressure with choking on his food.

Nutritional Needs—Milk
Is Still Most Important

Meanwhile, remember that the table bits are important only in keeping him interested in his food. At this age, his focus will be on feeding himself. If you keep feeding him because you fear he won't "eat enough," you can begin to set up resistance to the food you offer him. It's not worth it. Keep in his good graces. Milk is still the most important food that you give him.

10 Months

Too Busy Standing Up

Feeding times are becoming a circus. Mothers of 10-month-olds tell me that they are frustrated by their babies' attempts to stand up when they're supposed to be sitting down to eat. Your baby won't stay in his chair without trying out his new ability to stand! You'll have to be sure to strap him into the high chair (be sure it's been safety approved and follow the instructions that come with it) and stay right nearby. Otherwise he's very likely to stand up, turn around to hang on to its back, then topple over onto the floor.

Feeding now needs to become ritualized. That means using the same safe high chair with a strap to hold him in securely at each meal. One of the rituals your baby can expect at each meal is bits of food that you have ready to encourage him to eat—when he's hungry enough to want to participate. All this will help him learn to expect that meals always happen at the same time, in the same place, and in the same way. You'll need this routine to help settle him down. Feeding him in front of the television, however, is not a routine to set up. (See *Television and Eating Habits* in Chapter Three.)

Food Preferences

There may be more trouble to come. This period is the beginning of food preferences. One mother confided desperately, "He won't eat what I've gone to the trouble to fix for him. He just tastes it, shakes his head 'no,' and then pushes it aside and won't eat it. I could kill him!"

"Why is it so important to you that he eat it?" I asked.

"I go to so much trouble to make him a nice meal. When he won't take what I've made him, I feel like he's rejecting me! And anyway, I want him to have a rounded diet! He hardly lets me feed him any longer!"

To respond to these three passionate concerns, we offer the following suggestions:

1. Don't go to any extra trouble to prepare your child's food if this will make you take his refusal personally. A baby this age will be more interested in the same old routines and tastes. You may need to offer the same new food ten or fifteen times before he decides to try it.

2. A 10-month-old is headed toward the time when many babies won't accept a well-rounded diet. Milk and vitamins will help supplement what he will eat. Rather than fretting, or pressuring—which won't help—you should talk with your pediatrician to be sure that your baby's growth is on track and that he is getting all the nutrients (including iron) he needs.

3. You are about to be pushed away as a nurturer. I'd urge you to respect his need to be more independent in the feeding area and to set up his feedings so you can enjoy the steps he takes toward self-feeding. Otherwise, you may be headed toward food battles that you aren't likely to win.

4. Feed him foods of different textures and different tastes that he can pick up to master by himself. But introduce them often, and without pressure. Don't expect him to try them the first, second, or even the third time!

Avoiding Allergies

Eggs had better be saved until this age or later. Try egg yolk first, then, at about 12 months, egg whites. Scrambled eggs are great finger foods! But eggs are among the foods most likely to set off allergies in the form of skin rashes. Stop them right away if they do. Your doctor can then help you decide whether the rash is truly an allergic reaction, so that you won't have to give up on such a good source of protein unless you have to. If there is an allergy, avoid foods that contain eggs until well into the second year, when you will want to ask your doctor about whether to try them out again.

Breastfeeding

It is still to the baby's advantage to be on breast milk and to have the antibodies and digestive enzymes it provides. By now, though, other foods must provide some nutrients, especially iron and vitamin D, and eventually zinc. But breastfeeding can still be a lovely way for a mother and baby to bond again when the mother returns home at the end of the day. At this age, a mother may feel that her baby is so busy that he won't suck very long. She may worry that he isn't getting enough milk in the shortened feedings. But he will. In the first 5 minutes of feedings from a full breast, he can get as much as 6 ounces!

If your baby is bottle-fed, you can see and measure the same thing. He has become so efficient that he can wolf down 6 ounces in 8 minutes.

Time to Wean?

Should your baby be weaned now to a cup? I don't think so. A cup, or a sippie cup, can certainly be introduced. But a baby this age still needs a lot of sucking. Sucking is such a sure way of helping him learn to calm himself down when he is excited, and a wonderful way for him to handle the overload of a busy day. Sucking helps him settle down to a relaxed, sleepy state. It is a first strategy for him to learn to use to manage frustration, fatigue, excitement, and other overwhelming feelings.

I don't feel that sucking in a warm, cozy, cuddled situation should be given up in this first year. It's much too challenging a year. There is so much to be learned. Why should a baby be ready to give it up at 10 months?

Many mothers may be feeling ready to stop breastfeeding by now. But before making your decision, you may want to remember one mother we described earlier. She felt that each of the steps in this period of her baby's development seemed to be saying that her baby no longer needed her. But of course he does. And feeding is such a precious time to renew these lovely, warm feelings between you.

Let him practice all his new skills—finger feeding, using a cup, spoon, hands, refusals, pushing food over the edge of his high chair, trying to stand, saying words, and trying new uses of his mouth and vocal cords. All of these can be explored at a feeding. But consider continuing to breastfeed as a way to balance all of these new steps toward independence with the closeness that you both still need.

Transition to Mealtimes

You are setting the stage for mealtimes to be times for reunion and for your child to feel that food and eating are up to him. Over time, you both will feel ready to give up the closeness of breastfeeding when sharing other kinds of communication can begin to replace these delicious times together. As he learns to sit still and to feed himself and shares his early words with you, meals taken as a family can become an enjoyable time for closeness to replace the intimate cuddling possible with breastfeeding.

12 to 24 Months

1 Year Old!

A birthday cake with a single candle—and maybe one for good luck! A smear of icing over the face, hands, furniture, mom's dress, dad's jacket—who cares! It is so exciting to mark the accomplishments of that first, exciting year. Joyful parents are bound to feel, "We figured it out! We are parents now, and we have proven it!" Grandparents, aunts, uncles, cousins may secretly smirk at the big deal parents make of this event. Older siblings feel jealous and try to steal the first birthday thunder. But there's no way they really can. Few events match the momentousness of this milepost.

Parents are facing a turbulent year. They may have already sensed glimmerings. Parents in most cultures that raise feisty, independent children like we do will face a surge of independence and the beginning of defiance in this next year. The expression "the terrible twos" usually refers to this year and the next. If we could change the label to "the terrific twos," we might turn our expectations around. A toddler is learning so much, and he conveys such wonderful evidence of his learning. In the next two years he will begin to become independent, and feeding is one of the areas where this becomes clear. But eating patterns may also change because children's bodies grow more slowly now than during the first year of life, so they'll need less food than parents expect.

Fostering Independent Feeding

At 1 year, a child will be at an important crossroads for feeding. He will have learned that he can play with food or he can eat it. He can feed himself or he can feed the floor. He can make choices. He can shut his mouth tight. His opposition to being fed by others may be intense or mild. But no longer need he be at the mercy of being fed.

As parents, we need to recognize the opportunity we have at each feeding to enjoy and foster this independence, while keeping our role as protectors and nurturers. Can we accept the difference between the nurturing role we played when the child was "our baby" and the one we need to play now? As one mother said to me with tears in her eyes, "I hate giving up my baby. I know I want him to grow up, but I already feel as if I've lost him somehow. My only way to hold on to him is to be sure of his feeding. When he refuses me on that, too, I really feel as if my days of enjoying being a mother are over. It's no fun any longer."

A toddler demands that a parent face this new role. When a parent asks, "What do I do to stop a temper tantrum?" I have to break the news: "Nothing." When a parent asks, "How can I get him to eat a rounded diet?" again I must answer: "You can't." It hurts, doesn't it? It is so hard to let go and let a young child begin to learn on his own, especially when only he can help himself, and you *really* can't.

Ghosts from the Nursery

When I asked the mother of a 1-year-old baby, "Can you put up with his finger feeding and his playing with food?" she confided, "My stomach tightens up when he throws his food to the dog." "Do you have any idea why?" I asked.

"I hate to see food wasted," she said, unconvincingly.

"We all do, but I wonder why it gets to you so much," I persisted.

"Well, I can remember my own mother saying, 'You have to eat a little bit of everything. Clean your plate. There are children starving all over the world. You are lucky to have this food. You can't get up until you've finished your plate.'"

"Wow, that's quite a lot to remember," I said. "Do you think it has anything to do with your tightening stomach?"

She winced. "I swore I'd *never, ever* be like that with my children. I don't really want to be. What can I do?"

I try to help parents like this establish an alternative plan to help them face the 1-year-old's predictable opposition at mealtimes:

- Don't hover over him to feed him. Often, doing chores nearby in the kitchen keeps you out of it.
- Let him make his own choices.
- Offer two bits of finger food at a time, while you do your own work around the kitchen.
- Let him try out familiar and unbreakable utensils. Most children should be successful in using a spoon by 16 months. (In Japan, children begin to master chopsticks by 18 months! To me, this represents a toddler's determination to imitate his elders and to achieve a difficult step.)
- When he's downed two bits of food, give him two more.
- Stay behind him, not ahead of him in offering food.
- Try offering him one food at a time so he can concentrate on it without being distracted by others.
- When he begins to play with the food or throw it around, that's a signal: It's the end of the meal. Put him down calmly, and without criticism tell him, "All done."
- No food between meals other than at regular times for snacks. Snacks are necessary for young children. At regular times every day they can include part of the child's daily dietary requirements. But no grazing. Grazing is a parent's way of trying to slip food in when a child isn't paying attention. And it prevents a child from becoming hungry enough to sit down for a meal.

When you have your family meal, the baby can be in his high chair as long as he's focused on eating his food or contributing to the family's fun of being together. When he's not, and begins to tease and test, put him down and let him play somewhere else—where it is safe for him to be on his own.

I used to recommend that the whole family always eat together. But with my own family I soon found out what every parent of a toddler already knows: "It is hell having him at the table when all he does is tease you about food." If family meals are painful with a 1-year-old, let the child stay nearby so that mealtime remains a social time. This way you can keep your 1-year-old from connecting negative memories with mealtimes, making it harder for meals to be enjoyable even when he is older. Parents may do best to feed a baby this age before the family meal. Then, at family mealtimes, the baby's contribution can be purely social.

"But," a parent will say, "he won't eat enough that way. He plays with his food, and all he wants is his milk. He isn't good enough with a spoon or fork. He throws a cup around." Right. He senses how important food is to us as parents. To take pressure off parents, I focus on four elements of a toddler's diet that are necessary. I share them with a toddler's parents so they can be as relaxed as possible about how much a toddler needs to eat in a 24-hour period to grow and be healthy. The following foods can be spread out over three meals and two or three snacks each day. (Of course, each child's actual requirements will depend on a variety of individual factors, including size, activity, and metabolism, among others, so check with your pediatrician to be sure you know what *your* baby's nutritional needs are.)

Nutritional Needs in the Second Year
(Exact Amounts Vary from Child to Child)

1. 16 ounces of milk (necessary for calcium and protein)—either in two or three breast feedings or in two bottles of "follow-up" formula (formula with a different balance of nutrients adjusted for this age group). Follow-up formula should contain iron and vitamin D. Before a child is 1 year old, cow's milk is not recommended, as it contains little iron and may interfere with iron absorption. When a child is ready for cow's milk (check with your pediatrician), be sure it is whole milk and fortified with vitamin D. A cup of yogurt or an ounce or two of cheese can substitute for a serving of milk, as can chocolate milk or ice cream. The fat in whole milk dairy products contribute to brain development in the first years. If your child doesn't take milk or milk products for a while, ask his physician for a substitute for the calcium and vitamin D requirements.

2. Three to 4 ounces of protein. For example, a patty of cooked lean hamburger, an egg, beans, or tofu.

3. Half a slice of whole-grain bread and half a cup of whole-grain cereal, macaroni, or noodles should provide enough carbohydrates (along with the milk) as fuel for a child's active energy needs. By age 2, a child may need a little more. Whole grains will provide fiber to help prevent constipation.

4. Iron—meats such as hamburger also supply iron. Vegetables that contain iron (such as chick peas, lentils, baked beans,

(continued on next page)

Nutritional Needs in the Second Year
(continued from previous page)

spinach, and kale, among others) can be substituted, although the iron in them is less readily absorbed. (Give foods rich in vitamin C, such as cantaloupe, tomatoes, or citrus fruits, to enhance absorption.) But many children will balk at vegetables. If this is a difficult requirement, ask for iron drops from your child's doctor.

5. One or two pieces of fruit (before a baby turns one, citrus fruits are more likely to cause allergic skin rashes) or 3–4 ounces of fruit juice for vitamin C. Six ounces a day is the upper limit for children ages 1 to 6. Juice can cause cavities, and can fill a baby up before he's eaten the foods he really needs.

6. Try a variety of cooked vegetables or leafy greens, but don't push them. Don't assume your child will hate them, but don't be alarmed if he does. A relaxed attitude is the best away to prevent struggles and promote—gradually—a broad range of tastes. For now, though, a liquid multivitamin supplement with minerals given in drops can be used in the place of vegetables if your child won't eat them.

To prevent choking, watch out for fruit with pits or seeds, stringy vegetables like celery, and hard nuts and candies. Meat should be minced into small bits. With these main ingredients or their substitutes as a goal, most parents can relax and leave feedings to the child. Try to maintain the closeness that a milk feeding establishes at the end of each meal. Whether breastfeeding or bottle-feeding, continue to hold him, to cuddle him, to rock and croon to him. It's an important balance to his struggle for independence.

I do not recommend that children feed themselves a bottle—either during the day, or at night. A propped bottle or a bottle he carries around to feed himself is no substitute for the opportunity for communication at feeding time. When I see a child who carries his milk around with him, I think of three things:

1. How forlorn he looks.
2. How urgently his parent must feel about "getting milk into him." But he's missing the warmth that each feeding deserves, which can continue into this independent year. Save the bottle for times when you and he can be together.
3. Children who carry their bottles around with them and have access to them at all times are at risk of "bottle baby tooth decay"—baby teeth (especially upper front and molar teeth) full of cavities—and a greater risk of later cavities.

Nighttime Bottles

Leaving a bottle in bed with a child at night "to get enough milk in" is no better. *Before* settling a child in bed, a nighttime bottle or a last cozy breastfeeding can be used as a "lovey" to help him prepare for separation and sleeping. But if parents put a child to bed with a bottle of milk or juice, they are endangering the baby's future teeth. After a milk feeding at night, always give him water to clean out his mouth and protect his teeth from decay.

When and How to Wean

"All that is good is not forever." Nursing in the second year is not encouraged in our mainstream culture. In many other cultures, though, a child is weaned only when the mother becomes pregnant again. I admire a mother who dares to continue despite the pressures of our society. Mothers who are working outside the home have the additional challenge of pumping, bringing home milk, and maintaining their supply.

If a mother wants to breastfeed in the second year, she may find it helpful to consider her own reasons. It's not easy to breastfeed when a baby becomes a toddler. If a mother is breastfeeding because she finds it hard to give up her baby to a toddler's independence, she needs to be aware of this. A toddler's independence is the baby's most important job in the second year. If his mother can't tolerate his new challenges during this period, she may be interfering with these important new tasks.

But if you and your toddler are using continued breastfeeding for closeness, soothing, and nutritional reasons, you can enjoy these times while they last. You can even talk to the baby in simple terms about the feelings you both have during breastfeeding. At the same time, praise him for his feistiness to acknowledge his struggle for independence.

Weaning a child late in the second or third year can become more and more difficult, especially when a parent has mixed feelings about stopping. One way to help with the transition is to encourage use of a "lovey"—a substitute for the breast or bottle, something soft and comforting to touch, for example, a stuffed animal or a blanket. Tell him to go get his lovey when you are getting ready for a feeding. "Hug it while we nurse." Gradually emphasize the lovey as a way to comfort himself—when he falls or hurts himself, when he's making a difficult transition, such as going off to daycare or to bed. After a while, try to leave out a feeding and offer him the lovey instead.

If he has been in the habit of fingering your hair or your other breast, he may turn to his own skin or hair to soothe himself. Good for him! It makes weaning an easier transition, and he'll be learning to rely on himself for self-comforting.

You can still offer him the bedtime nursing "for comfort" even if you haven't much milk. Offer him a little water before bed after any milk or solid feeding—to help avoid tooth decay. Even if you've stopped these last feedings, sit by him at bedtime, so he won't feel that no more breastfeeding means he's losing you. Remind him that he has already learned to comfort himself with his lovey. You are turning over responsibility to settle himself for sleep to him. Gradually, he'll be able to turn to the lovey. But don't resort to leaving him with a bedtime bottle.

As you wean him, emphasize the cup. Be sure to offer plenty of dairy products—cheese, yogurt, and ice cream as well as milk in a cup (or in a bottle during the day). Cow's milk is safe for most children over 1 year of age. The fat in whole milk is important for brain development at least until age 2.

Mothers must decide when weaning is appropriate from their point of view, but their child's behavior can be their guide. Weaning seems important for the child's sake when everyone around him begins to disapprove. He will take it personally. A child may feel, "I'm too much of a baby." At that point, continued breast-feeding may be endangering his self-esteem. Don't let it.

When to Wean from Bottle Feeding

Just as with weaning from the breast, find him a lovey that he can use whenever he needs it. I'd urge you to choose one that no one will disapprove of if he needs it for several years—a bear

---

How to Handle High Chair Struggles

Q: How do you feed a child who struggles and fights whenever you want to put him in his high chair?

A: Be as firm and definite as you can be: "Now it's time for your supper." Cut down on competing stimuli (send older children out of the room). Offer him an attractive object related to feeding—a teething biscuit, a cracker, whatever he happens to like at the time, but nothing sugary if possible. (Once you start with sweets as a reward, your child may resist eating anything else.)

Q: When he struggles to get out of his high chair, what do I do? He's just learning to walk and I know he's excited about it.

A: Try to make feeding an expected ritual: "It's time to eat." Use the protective strap or belt on his seat to hold him, and offer a bit of food he likes. When he's too resistant, forget about food. Put him down until the next meal.

Q: Should I feed him while he's walking around?

A: No. Feedings should be a ritual. Feeding him without sitting him down could lead to grazing and might interfere with his learning to tell when he is hungry and when he's had enough. He will be even less likely to sit in his high chair.

or a blanket, or even a truck. Encourage him to hold and stroke it as he drinks from his bottle. Then, gradually, wean him from the bottle to the lovey. Promise him a bottle at mealtimes and *before* bedtimes. Then gradually cut down to the lovey. It may take a month. Be patient.

A Meal Plan in the Second Year

Three well-balanced meals is ideal—containing, for example, minced meat or hamburger, mashed potatoes, rice, or pasta, and carrots or green vegetables if you don't have to struggle to get your child to eat them, apple sauce or a piece of fruit for desert, juice (no more than 4–6 ounces a day), plus two regularly scheduled snacks (some crackers, yogurt, cheese, or cut up fruits and vegetables). If the child eats well at mealtimes, a snack in the morning and one in the evening should usually be enough.

The average daily energy allowance for 1-year-olds is 98 calories per kilogram of weight, or roughly 850 calories per day. But the actual number of calories a child needs will vary not only with his size, but also his metabolism, his activity level, and other individual factors. Check with your doctor if your child seems to be gaining too much or too little weight. At 12 months, normal weight can range from about 17 to 28 pounds and height (length) from 27 to 32 inches. At age 2, normal weight can range from 23 to 33 pounds and height from 31 to 37 inches (according to the National Center for Health Statistics, 2000).

Learning to Drink from a Cup

You can introduce your baby to a cup when he is 6 or 7 months old, and expect him to drink from it as you hold it by 9 months. But he probably won't be able to drink from a cup on his own until about 12–15 months. Even then, be prepared for spills. Sippie cups can certainly help. Gaily decorated ones will motivate children who are slow to make this transition.

After our children had their first taste of bath water in a cup, we started to put a little bit of milk or fruit juice in their cups at mealtimes. Usually, though, our dog, Alice, got more of the milk than any of our children did. She had already been alerted to such opportunities by the food on the floor at the end of each meal. Although Alice spent most of her time sprawled out asleep in the front hall, she was always ready for mealtimes. I can remember the glow on our oldest daughter's face when she realized that she could share her food with the dog!

2- and 3-Year-Olds

At ages 2 and 3, a child is beginning not only to be independent but to become aware of himself and of other's feelings. He is building a self-image. Some children may be hungry to try everything out on their own but are not yet able to achieve the independence they are fighting for. By listening to the child, parents can support this fabulous pursuit for understanding self and others.

In the first year, feeding and food have been established as one important form of communication between a child and his parents. As a result, he knows these are important. But feeding times will also become times for the play that is the young child's most important way of learning about his world. Hunger is overshadowed by the passion behind these quests. A parent of a toddler may well feel daunted by the child's intense drive to use food and mealtimes for play and learning. Parents are equally passionate about making sure their child is nourished. But they won't win any battle they set up in this arena.

Food Play

When a 2-year-old piles his finger food up into a tower, then knocks it down to spray the room, it may seem that he does it to anger his parents. When he drops bits of food over one side of his tray, then another, and then a third, parents will certainly feel hurt that his food did not end up in his mouth.

When a 3-year-old calls your attention to the "picture" he has made out of bright orange carrots and green beans, he is demonstrating his new words and his new awareness of the beauty of colors as he arranges them side by side. He is using food to test his new skills. To a parent it feels like teasing or making a mess with important, hard-earned ingredients: "I went to a lot of trouble to cook those two vegetables for him—carrots and beans. All he wants to do is play with them." His mother is missing the other appeals that these two vegetables offer him—colors and textures.

Ghosts from Earlier Generations

At many times in the past and in many cultures, food has meant survival. As if to teach a generation that has not known hunger, parents or grandparents may remind children about starving children elsewhere in the world who would love to finish up what they won't eat. Of course, no one ever does wrap up the leftovers to send to hungry children—even though there are all too many, and not just on the other side of the world. The child senses that parents are pressuring him, and the message can complicate a child's attitude toward eating.

My own parents were second-generation Texas settlers. They were steeped in the struggles of their parents to make a living in this new land and to provide food for their families. Food was too precious to be played with. I can remember my mother's stern face when I left food on my plate, or when I refused it. I found that I couldn't avoid replaying my mother's strong feelings with my own children. When they seemed to be "playing with their food," for example, I had to learn not to comment on it. But still, I was haunted by my mother's disapproving glare when I refused to eat.

Should a parent give in to the child's need to play with food, and let him tease? I don't think so. Although it's easier said than done, parents can make it clear that food is for eating, not play. But making an issue of it will only lead to even more creative food activities. When a child has begun to play with his food and has lost interest in eating it, simply remove his plate and tell him, "All done" or "It looks like you've finished eating. Did you like it?" Then, remove him from the table and let him settle down to play on his own. Simply stopping the behavior in this firm but gentle way will be far more effective than criticizing or punishing it. Eventually he will understand that the reward of staying at the table with the family depends on his learning to feed himself the way everyone else does. He will be far more motivated to imitate adult table manners if punishments are not associated with mealtimes.

There is a well-known study in which toddlers were allowed to choose their own foods over a period of several months. Observers kept records of their choices. Over that extended period, the children balanced their diet with all the ingredients necessary for optimal growth. Leaving such choices to children two, three, and four is tough! But it is easier when parents recognize that all they have now is control over the range of food choices that are offered.

Strategies for Feeding 2- and 3-Year-Olds

- Set up the feeding situation as a time for the child to be in control as much as possible. This means that eating with others who will be likely to tell the child what to do is not a good choice.
- A toddler may need to be fed alone—not isolated, but fed at a time and place where food and his choices are not the focus.
- If your child seems distracted when you sit down to be with him during his meals, do your own chores around the kitchen to take pressure off him while he eats.
- When he becomes ready for it (around age 2 or so) sit down with the child while he eats, as long as food is not the subject. You and others who won't comment on his eating can keep him company so that he can learn to look forward to mealtimes as a time to enjoy being together.

(continued on next page)

Strategies for Feeding 2- and 3-Year-Olds
(continued from previous page)

- Use a child-safe booster seat, securely fastened.
- Use a sippie cup, and don't fill it too much. Expect spills.
- The child's bowl should be anchored by suction to his tray.
- Don't make special foods for him if you will be disappointed when he refuses them or plays with them.
- Plan to give him more nourishing foods first, while he is most likely to be hungry: protein-containing foods (such as meat, cheese, and eggs), fruits or vegetables, and sips of milk from his cup. Whole-grain bread or crackers, or pasta, which are also important, are often more appealing to young children, so offer them later. Save sweets for dessert.
- Continue to offer only two bits of food at a time, then two more, until he begins to drop them or throw them.
- Don't expect him to chew his foods. You may find hunks in his stool. Don't worry. He'll absorb what he needs.
- Don't expect him to be excited by new or different foods. Children at this age are often put off by new foods. Instead, they'll find ways to make the "same old" foods seem interesting to them.
- "Manners" come later—at ages 4 and 5, but not now. Messiness is to be expected.
- Blowing food or throwing it is a pastime. Be prepared and decide ahead of time about the limits you'll set. Then, without excitement, say, "That's the end of the meal" and put him down.
- Ignore his requests for grazing between meals. This will be the hardest if he hasn't eaten "enough." Relax about a "balanced diet" if the child is healthy and growing. Over time, if struggles over food have been avoided, children will eat what they need—as long as it is offered to them.
- Punch some pillows or call a friend if you need to work off some frustration. Parents need each others' support at times like these.

Frequently Asked Questions
About Feeding 2- and 3-Year-Olds

Q: My toddler is so pokey when it comes to eating. I don't know whether he's just being negative or not. When do I stop the meal and put him down?

A: Let a pokey eater poke. Plan to have other things to do to distract yourself. If necessary, set a time limit and put him down after you've reached it. Next time, he may be more motivated to eat.

Q: My toddler won't eat any green foods one week, and then the next, he won't eat any yellow ones. Should I worry about his pickiness?

A: No. He's testing his ability to make choices. You may have trouble keeping up with his choice making but don't get too excited about it. He probably enjoys the experience of leading you around by the nose. I suggest that you present him with a limited choice of healthy foods at each meal and snack, including some that you know he's likely to eat. Then the choice is his. If he rejects them all, calmly let him know that "this is what we're having for supper today. If there isn't anything on the table that interests you, then maybe you'll like what we're having tomorrow better." It should be clear that there is no punishment involved. Instead, mealtimes are a chance to be together and make choices from the foods that are offered. Period. Don't jump up and cater to his requests, unless you want him to become accustomed to ordering you around. (See *Weaning* in *12 to 24 Months.*)

4- and 5-Year-Olds

Identifying with Adults
By age 4, a child is aware of his effect on others. He measures himself against the world around him, and he wants to be like the adults he admires. When a child this age identifies with adults and imitates them, he is ready to begin learning about table manners. They won't come all at once. Patience, practice, encouragement, and repetition will be needed for him to master them. But he'll also need you to model table manners and healthy eating habits!

Imitation
Watch for the effect of this modeling on a child's mealtime behaviors. He begins to hold a fork like his father or spears a slippery vegetable like his mother. He sits up to the table like one of his parents. He may even begin to eat vegetables. He even tries to cut his meat. But none of this is easy. The meat slips off his plate. "Oops! Daddy, can you cut it for me?" The cost of failure makes him regress. Then he teases. He spills his milk. He pushes his vegetables off his plate. He falls apart. But he has tried to live up to his parents.

Next time, he'll get even further in identifying with his parents. Or he'll find another way. An older sibling can become a model. If an older brother plays at the table, so will he. If siblings want a second helping, so will he. If a brother or sister eats green and yellow vegetables, he may too. If they display even a semblance of table manners, so will he. Commend him for his efforts. Rather than picking on what he doesn't do, try emphasizing what he does do. Offer to cut up his food, but be prepared and respectful if he wants to manage it for himself. If he can't, cut it up in the kitchen next time.

Picky Eating and Food Refusal

These years are times for children to get into eating like the rest of the family—vegetables, using utensils rather than fingers, using a napkin rather than a bib, manners, sitting on a booster chair. But it is also a time when rebellion can take over. "No milk—just juice." "I'll wait for dessert." Only green vegetables—or yellow or red or no vegetables. A 4- or 5-year old is likely to use fingers, pickiness, or refusals to establish his independence or to play out his conflicts. Expect it and don't get into it with him except to acknowledge it: "You seem like you've really made up your mind about those green beans. There'll be other things to try tomorrow."

What can a parent do? I would suggest that a parent ignore the child's bid for a struggle as much as possible. If the child continues to dominate the family's time together, maybe it's time for that child to be excused from the table—until the next meal. Being ignored may be the most effective discipline for a child this age who is setting up a struggle over food.

Hold your line on the choices. "Juice in the morning, milk at every meal." Try to ignore his fixed interest in always eating certain foods and let him have them, unless they are unhealthy.

Children this age are usually not interested in change or in trying out new foods. Their task at this age is learning table manners, starting with sitting still, using forks, knives, and spoons, eating and drinking without spills, and participating in mealtime conversation.

Keep junk food out of the house. "But other kids have them" is no excuse for junk food. Stand your ground and answer simply, "That's fine. You can try all that stuff when you visit." There is no point in making a fuss about an occasional taste of junk food at a friend's house—the more you make of it, the more appealing it is likely to become for your child. Over time, your child can even learn to be proud of his healthy choices and sophisticated tastes. Most of all, your child will learn to appreciate the foods that are present in his home, on his kitchen table—the foods that he sees his parents eat.

Food refusal can be a 4- or 5-year-old's way of establishing independence. Binges, pickiness, apparent "addictions" to one food and refusal of another are common at this age. Getting attention at the table and enlisting siblings in the struggle are also a part of this thrust toward independence.

Parents need to decide ahead of time how they will handle dessert. If dessert is only for children who have "finished" eating, food becomes a reward for good behavior instead of a source of nutrition and pleasure. It's easier to maintain healthy attitudes toward food and to avoid struggles if everyone has dessert when it is "dessert time." Desserts come after meals and are just that—the conclusion of a meal, not a reward, and not offered separately. Desserts that are particularly sweet and rich (for example, junk food pastries) are especially likely to interfere with a child's concentration on the rest of the meal—unless they are an unexpected surprise. Be sure that your desserts are not too exciting and are nourishing enough to make up for food shoved aside to "save room" for dessert. Fruit, applesauce, yogurt, and oatmeal cookies with nuts and raisins are possibilities.

A parent might say, "If you're not going to eat any more of your food, you may leave the table. Dessert? No, that's for when we're all ready." But remember that food can easily lose its value compared with the child's need to establish himself. At this age, his main struggle is to stand his ground and to save face. Your response needs to respect that as his most important goal.

When to Worry

Any prolonged refusal of more than a few kinds of foods may be a deeper cry for help. It may be a time to consider what is behind it. "Is he ill?" is a first question. Look for other signs. Have him weighed to see whether his general health is endangered. Consult with his doctor or nurse to rule out a medical problem. He may need a therapeutic evaluation so you and he can understand what's behind this behavior. (See *Food Refusal* in Chapter Three.)

Mealtimes as Social Times

In busy families, breakfast, dinner, and weekend meals may be the main opportunities to be together. But pressure to "please eat this, dear" can turn children against family meals and against eating. Be sure the table is a place for family talk—not punishment or pressure.

Family mealtimes can teach children so many things—for example, to recognize hunger cues and feeling "full," to appreciate the effort that has gone into preparing food, and to enjoy the pleasure of eating together. Sharing food, ideas, traditions, and conversation become memorable to any child. If started early, and protected from intrusions and outside pressures, meals together will become a family's most important time for communicating and showing deep caring for each other.

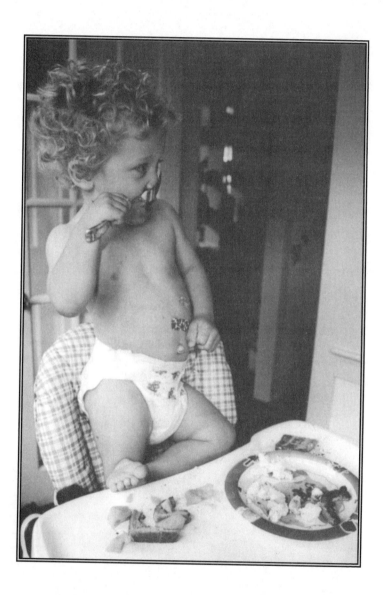

CHAPTER 3

Feeding Problems and Solutions

Allergies to Foods

Infancy is the best time to identify a child's allergic responses to foods. It is easier to do this then, because you can carefully introduce one food at a time. A skin rash—often appearing first on the face or in the creases of the arms, legs, and neck—that develops into a dry, scaly skin condition called eczema is a sign of an allergic reaction. Such rashes need to be taken seriously.

Reactions to cow's milk may show up even before solids are started, most often at 4 to 6 months of age. Food allergies can also begin with the introduction of solids. Start with only one at a time, so that if your baby does develop an allergic reaction such as a skin rash, you'll know which food caused it. Start with a simple cereal—rice, for example. No mixtures. Give the baby a two-week trial before introducing another solid. Then try fruit or vegetables, one at a time. Check the labels of baby food containers to be sure there are no other ingredients or additives. Save the introduction of wheat until 7 months, when you can give your baby a crust of bread to hold and to suck on. Save egg yolk until at least 10 months. Egg whites come even later—around 1 year of age. Wheat and eggs are more likely to cause allergies if given earlier. When basic foods must be avoided, be sure your pediatrician considers vitamin and mineral supplements (such as iron and vitamin D) and helps you plan a balanced diet for your infant. She or he will also decide with you whether and when (sometimes at 12 or 24 months) it is safe to try out a particular food again to see if your baby has outgrown the allergy.

A peanut allergy may last a lifetime, and can cause particularly severe reactions. Peanuts and peanut butter are not safe for children under age 3 in any event, because they can cause choking. Peanut products, including peanut oil, which is present in so many foods, are more likely than many other foods to cause allergies if eaten before this age.

If your baby does develop signs of a food allergy during the two weeks after you've introduced a new food, eliminate it. Keep a record of all foods that have caused allergic reactions. Later, if your child develops eczema or asthma, you'll want to keep her away from any foods that have caused allergic reactions. When you add other stresses, such as a bad cold or a bad pollen day, an acute asthma attack may result.

If you can eliminate foods that have caused only mild allergic reactions, this combined effect may not occur. It is important to pay attention to these reactions early, when the child's diet is not as complicated as it will be later. Food additives and mixtures of different foods should be avoided, because when a child does develop an allergic reaction, they make it harder to know exactly what caused it.

Certain foods (for example gluten-containing foods) or food additives to which a child may be sensitive have been thought by some to contribute to hyperactivity and other symptoms similar to those of attention-deficit hyperactivity disorder (ADHD). If so, then there may also be an underlying vulnerability to such symptoms. (See *Resources.*)

Bedtime Bottles

Many children need a "lovey," something to hold onto to take the place of parents at times of separation such as going to sleep at night. Some babies become accustomed to using the breast or bottle this way, falling asleep with one or the other still in their mouths. Putting them to sleep by breastfeeding or with a bottle is an easy pattern to fall into.

But milk in the baby's mouth can cause baby teeth to decay and can even increase the risk of tooth decay for permanent teeth later on. *Never* put a baby to bed with milk, juice, or anything but water (no sugar) in her bottle. If you feed a baby at bedtime, give her water afterward. If she's consuming enough milk for her age, she doesn't need a nighttime bottle for nutrition. She's using it to calm down. If she needs her bottle as a "lovey" to cuddle with at night, give her an empty one or one with water. Offer her a stuffed animal or a blanket to fondle at bottle times. Wean her gradually. Later, she'll be able to rely on this "lovey" rather than the bottle to settle at night.

Choking

Choking is a major cause of death in infants and young children. There are many ways to prevent choking, and parents can be prepared to help.

Foods That Can Cause Choking

Children 3 and under are at risk of choking on small nonfood items as well as on food. A number of foods are especially likely to cause choking and should be avoided. These are either small, hard, round foods that can block the young child's small windpipe or semisolid or sticky foods that can get stuck on the way down. For children 3 years old and under, avoid hard candies and gum balls, peanuts and other nuts, fruits with pits or large seeds (for example, cherries and watermelon) unless the pits and seeds are removed, raw carrots and celery, peanut butter, hunks of meat, and hot dogs. The risk of choking can also be lowered by feeding a child only when she is safely seated and not on the run.

How to Handle Choking

Before your child has a choking episode, read a guide to infant CPR (such as the *Children's Hospital Guide to Your Child's Health and Development*—see *Bibliography*). You may also want to take a CPR course from the Red Cross or a local hospital. Before 8 months, all parents will want to have instructions handy on maneuvers to help a choking baby. You'll be glad you're prepared.

If your child is able to cough up the food or object on her own, let her. If she can't give a good cough and is having trouble breathing, but is conscious, do the following: With an infant (under 1 year of age), face her belly down on your forearm, head down, supporting her head and neck firmly with your hand. With a heavy baby you many need to support that arm with your knees. With the heel of your other hand, hit her five times between the shoulder blades. If she still doesn't cough up the offending food or object, put your free hand and arm over her back and turn her over onto her back, supporting her head and neck, keeping her head below her body. Then press on the infant's chest, just below nipple level, but not at the bottom of her breastbone, up to five times with two or three fingers. Alternate these back blows and chest thrusts until the baby coughs up the piece of food or small object.

If your infant appears to be unconscious or not breathing, try to rouse her gently and then shake her shoulder. If she does not respond, shout for someone to call 911 for emergency help so that you can stay with your baby. If no one is nearby, make the call yourself, but keep your baby with you. In either case, then start infant CPR.

For a child over 1 year of age, who is conscious but cannot speak or cough, use the Heimlich maneuver first (see the *Children's Hospital Guide*). This maneuver isn't recommended for babies under 1 year. If a child over a year old appears to be unconscious after gently tapping her and then shaking her shoulder, call for help, stay with the child, and begin child CPR procedures. (After proper positioning, rescue breaths, repositioning, and another trial of rescue breaths, the Heimlich maneuver is another step in the CPR guidelines for unconscious children.)

Failure to Thrive

What Is Failure to Thrive?

Failure to thrive is a serious but not uncommon medical condition that usually begins during the first year of life. Affected children are below the fifth percentile in weight for age or have a slowed rate of weight gain. If the condition is not treated early and effectively, growth can be retarded, and poor nutrition can interfere with brain development.

What Causes Failure to Thrive?

Failure to thrive is a very general term that refers to babies and young children who are not eating or growing adequately. There are many reasons why this can happen. Some babies may appear to eat normally, but don't grow as they should. They may have a medical condition that interferes with the absorption of nutrients in their digestive system. Sometimes infections are the cause. There are many rarer medical conditions that can interfere with growth, including cystic fibrosis, sickle cell anemia, hypothyroidism, heart disease, kidney disease, and others.

Some babies with failure to thrive are not eating enough. They may have a hypersensitivity to taste or to touch in their mouths, a hypersensitive gag reflex that causes them to choke on food and make them afraid to eat, poor coordination of the tongue and throat muscles needed for swallowing, or gastroesophageal reflux (see *Spitting Up, Gastroesophageal Reflux, and Pyloric Stenosis* in this chapter).

There may also be psychological reasons underlying a baby's poor eating. Parent-infant interactions can affect and be affected by the infant's difficulties with eating. Though parents are bound to blame themselves, this is not likely to be anyone's fault. Eating problems may arise from a medical condition that a parent may not at first be aware of. For example, a baby with gastroesophageal reflux may come to connect feeding with the pain of acid reflux and the fear of gagging. She may start to refuse the bottle in order to avoid the pain. Parents, anxious to feed her, may add their tension to hers, or even try to force-feed her out of desperation. A vicious cycle is set up—and the baby will only fight off food all the more. When this occurs, the parents and the baby's physician need to work together as a team to defuse the struggle and help the child grow normally.

Because failure to thrive can be due to medical reasons, such as poor absorption or reflux of foods, reflux of food, a medical evaluation is necessary. Your pediatrician will check for infections, malabsorption syndromes, and other causes. She or he may even have the child spend a few days in the hospital. If none of these tests reveal any reason for poor nutrition and growth, you and your doctor will want to be sure that rarer possibilities are considered, such as those mentioned above.

Treatment of failure to thrive depends on the cause that is identified. Sometimes swallowing problems and oral hypersensitivity are subtle. Sometimes the child's fears, and the parents', have taken on a life of their own—causing serious interference with feeding. Often a team of professionals is needed—a pediatrician (sometimes a pediatric gastroenterologist), a nutritionist, even a speech specialist knowledgeable about the role of throat and mouth muscles in this disorder, and a mental health professional (social worker, psychologist, child psychiatrist) who can help the child and family overcome the patterns that have taken hold of feeding interactions. Parents will need to search for specially adapted ways of feeding their baby and to look to the baby to show them that these feeding interactions have become more comfortable.

Fathers and Feeding

Fathers are bound to feel left out as mothers nurse their babies. Their longing to be important to their new baby needs to be valued—though it may leave them feeling confused. They may not be aware that their fathers felt this way when they were being raised. For many fathers, the wish to nurture and to be nurtured isn't easily discussed.

Over the years, we have begun to recognize the positive effects of involved fathers on their children's development and the needs of fathers to be emotionally important and nurturing for their child. Just as women have come into their own in the workplace, men are discovering their need to take a more active role in nurturing. Men are more likely to be respected now for their commitment to nurturing their infants and children. Even so, most fathers still play only a secondary role when it comes to preparing food for and feeding children.

I would urge that a father be enlisted to feed the baby from the first. If the mother is trying to establish her breast milk supply, it may not be wise for him to feed the baby a bottle right away. But from the beginning he can participate by bringing the baby to the mother for feeding, along with some cushions to help her get comfortable. By about 3 weeks, when the mother's milk is established, a father can feed a bottle (with either expressed breast milk or formula) to the baby at night while the mother rests. This way, the baby can get used to two different kinds of sucking. Waiting much longer (4 to 6 weeks) may keep the baby from ever adjusting to the bottle.

Fathers who feed for the first time are likely to feel clumsy and tentative. So will the baby. She may already be used to working hard at the breast. She may gulp down her bottle-feeding, taking air with each noisy gulp. A wise father who hears his baby gulping will be prepared for forceful bubbles. Gingerly bubble her in the midst of the feeding, because the air underneath the milk can result in a sudden blast of milk and air. At the end of such a feeding, prop her at a 30 degree angle for 15–20 minutes before your final attempt at burping her. The milk will be more likely to stay down.

A first-time father needs to be protected from advice-giving observers: "That's not the way you hold a new baby! That's not the way you feed a baby!" No one can resist the urge to correct a new father. Be strong and be determined to try it out your own way. It's your baby, too! And you can and will learn so much from experimentation.

Learning about a baby is a process of trial and error. Mistakes are an inevitable part of finding a parent's way. But she'll be a lucky baby if her father learns about her and can feed her

---

What Fathers Add to Feeding

- A father is more likely to be playful and tease the baby at mealtimes: "Here! Reach out for the spoon with your mouth!" Or, as he directs a food-laden spoon toward the baby's mouth: "Open up! Here comes the airplane."
- He may hold a spoon differently and offer solids in a way that makes the baby learn two different ways of accepting and swallowing these solids.
- He will offer a cup and use one himself to help the baby learn by modeling.
- He may not be as concerned about "how much" the baby eats. This may lessen the pressure around mealtimes.
- When the child is at the family table, he can offer playful conversation and interesting topics. "Do you know what tigers like to eat?"
- A child who can keep her father involved at mealtimes is getting a boost to her self-image: "I'm important to him so I *am* important!"

too. Use a rocking chair. Cuddle your baby before and after the feeding. Put her out in front of you on your legs to talk to her and to admire her. She will get to know you that way.

A baby will choose her father's voice and face over another male's voice and face by 2 weeks of age. She is already working to know you. And by 2 months, she will know you as a unique person in her life. Continue to feed her regularly, so she knows your smell, your touch, your way of holding her, and your way of talking to her at feeding times.

A father should be an active participant in each of his child's touchpoints of feeding. Give your wife some relief by sharing responsibility for the baby's feedings. And give her the chance to express her feelings about sharing the baby with you. The baby will profit from your sharing. She will "know" each of you more intimately.

Food Shopping and Cooking with Children

When a child accompanies her parent to shop for food, she can learn so much. This can be an opportunity to share the customs of your family and of your culture. "We don't eat pork or bacon." "We need some rice to go with the beans." "We don't eat meat in our family." You can even help your child learn colors (of fruits and vegetables) and numbers ("How many cookies should we get?"). You can help her get ready to read during your visit to the grocery store. When you stop and read the labels to make your choices, your child learns about the power of the written word. She also learns that you pay close attention to the food you put in your body, and hers.

This can also be an opportunity to balance the effects of junk food advertising. Not by talking about junk food, but by making other foods more interesting. "We can make you a delicious sandwich with this nice fresh (whole wheat) bread." Or, "If we get peas in their pods and shell them together, they'll taste fresher than canned or frozen peas." Then let her compare tastes.

When she goes to the market with you, ask her to help look for the foods. "Can you help me find the tomatoes we like?" This can be an opportunity to explain which foods are best for her body, and why. What do they do? But keep it fun and respect her tolerance. Otherwise, food may become too serious, a burden instead of a pleasure. Be prepared for her to be ready to leave before you are. Bring a small toy or a book to distract her while you finish your shopping.

Do not use the candy at the checkout counter as a bribe. It sets a precedent. To the child, you may seem to be saying, "Whenever you want candy, just whine or throw a temper tantrum. It worked this time." Instead, you'd like her to know that "food shopping is a job we have to do. I need you to help me—so I can get your advice from time to time." Let her carry a small change purse and pick out a piece of fruit or crackers to pay for at the counter. This way she can learn about money, and will start to count change by the time she's 4 or 5.

Afterward, try to interest her in preparing food together. You can show an older child how to turn a pancake in the pan. (Be sure she knows never to cook unless you are right by her side.) Let her measure ingredients for a favorite recipe, or tear up lettuce, or slice a banana (with a dull knife that won't cut her). Start early with safe and simple ways to participate—at least by the time she is 2. Let her help you set the table. When dishes and utensils need to be cleared, she can be given this job. (Use plastic plates and cups.) The child then becomes part of a busy family's "work" and can learn to feel proud of her new ability to join in and help.

Food can help hold a family together. Children's participation from the first few years can give them a feeling of how rewarding teamwork in a family can be.

Food Refusal

Food refusal can take the form of a "hunger strike" lasting several days or re-emerging from time to time. Or certain foods at each meal may be refused—either the same ones each time or different ones. Sometimes food refusal can even include hiding, dumping, or throwing food—anything to avoid eating it. All this is upsetting to parents, who know that one of their most important responsibilities is to nourish their child.

What a child eats must be her choice. However, parents can set the stage for children's choices through the foods they choose to serve and by their own eating habits that they offer as a model. Although parents decide what and how much food to provide for the child at each meal, they can't force her to eat. What and how much she eats is inevitably up to her. Parents would do best to step back, as much as possible, as their child makes these decisions.

Although food refusal is likely to be due to the child's resistance to pressure from parents to eat, there are other possible causes. Among these are hypersensitivities to certain tastes and textures, a hypersensitive gag reflex, trouble swallowing leading to choking, or digestive system problems that lead a child to connect eating with pain. Any negative experiences that a child has with food, particularly strongly negative or repeated ones, can lead a child to avoid food. (See *Gag Reflex* and *Spitting Up, Gastroesophageal Reflux, and Pyloric Stenosis.*)

Children are bound to rebel against parental pressure to eat. This pressure can be obvious or subtle. Parents may not even be aware of it. Whether they are or not, parents' pressure will *never* work. I would urge parents to reconsider their own "ghosts from the nursery" about food, mealtimes, and eating and to handle these memories without involving the child. Otherwise they can become a source of unexpected food refusal. "Eat your vegetables—just one bite and you'll find you like them" or "See how Mommy eats her meal—you can grow up to be just like me—just eat what I do" or "Clean your plate!" All of these are better left unsaid.

During defiant periods (for example, the second and third years), meals can demand tolerance from parents. If parents are patient, by the age of 4, children will begin to model on their parents' manners, eating habits, and balanced food choices.

Gag Reflex and
Swallowing Problems

All babies gag when solid foods are first introduced at 4 to 6 months of age. Most will first push away the spoon with their tongues because of a reflex (the extrusion reflex) that is still active at this age. If they do this for several days in a row, they may be trying to tell you they're not ready for solids yet. Try again in a week or so to see if this reflex has become less reactive.

Some babies, though, gag and spit up even earlier, such as when a bottle is introduced. The gag reflex itself may be hypersensitive. Or the swallowing muscles may be poorly coordinated. Typically there are three components of sucking:

1. The lapping of the tongue in the front of the mouth
2. The massaging and pull from the back of the tongue
3. The pull from the throat

But in some babies these different actions are not working together. Each one is set off alone, and the separate movements don't come together to pull in your finger. In fact, your finger may set off an opposite reaction—vomiting or spitting up. If you find this happening, consult your child's doctor about ways to help the baby feed successfully.

Some babies' mouths and tongues may be especially hyper-sensitive—to touch, texture, or taste. When this is the case, it may help for you to press firmly on the baby's lips *before* you offer the finger or the feeding. You may even need to press with your finger on the insides of her cheeks and on her palate. Then the baby may begin to suck normally. But keep your finger away from the back of her throat, where you can set off the gag reflex and make her become more uncomfortable and spit up. (See *Spitting Up, Gastroesophageal Reflux, and Pyloric Stenosis.*)

Illnesses and Eating

When a child feels lousy, she won't want to eat. If she's vomiting, she'll refuse food and fluids. Dehydration is an immediate concern and can often be prevented. If she also has an upset stomach, temporarily stop her milk and solids. Resort to clear liquids with sugar and salts that she may need to replace. When she vomits repeatedly, try flat ginger ale, or fall back on a hydration solution: 1 tablespoon sugar and ½ teaspoon salt to 8 ounces of water. Give her 1 teaspoonful every 5–10 minutes at first. As she retains that, go to 1 tablespoon every 5 minutes the second hour. If she begins to vomit again, start over, and let your doctor know.

For an upper respiratory infection, such as a runny nose, cough, or flu, be sure she gets plenty of liquids. If her throat is sore, she may need more encouragement to drink. For an older child, either warm or cold drinks (even Popsicles) may be soothing. Offer her clear liquids every hour or so. Milk and solids may well seem too heavy, and she may refuse them.

When your child has diarrhea and vomiting, your main job is to keep her from becoming dehydrated by giving her plenty of fluids containing salts and sugars. If she has a fever too, fluids may also help bring her temperature down and give her enough energy to start eating again. You may have to use your ingenuity to get her to drink when she feels lousy. Even lollipops or salted crackers may help to make her thirsty.

Signs of Dehydration

- Fewer wet diapers or, in an older child, less frequent urination
- Dry skin, sunken eyes
- Dry mouth and tongue
- Lethargy and irritability
- Rapid pulse

If your child shows any of these signs or you have any reason to suspect that she is dehydrated, call your doctor right away.

If you need to clear a baby's nose so that she can suck and drink, you can either use nose drops diluted half and half with water before you try to feed her, or you can make up your own nose drops (½ teaspoon salt to 4 ounces of water). Use a few drops 10–15 minutes before you feed her.

Junk Food

Stacked high in supermarkets, convenience stores, and even drug stores and gas stations—and tempting your children as they wait in the checkout line—junk food is everywhere. It's in the fast food restaurants on the strip malls that have overtaken many neighborhoods, and it's on television, selling itself to your children. Junk food even masquerades as "healthy," "low-fat," and "all-natural" food.

What is a parent to do?

First, it helps to understand what you are up against. Our children's tastes are overwhelmed by the advertising they see on television. But you don't have to let them watch it! Rent videos, watch commercial-free stations, read books together to protect your child from being lured into the sugar, salt, and fat habits that come with soda pop, chips, candy, sweetened cereals, fast food burgers and pizzas. The average young child spends more time in front of the television than she does in school. Active sports and active play are being replaced by television viewing for many young children. Television-watching time should also be limited to prevent weight gain caused by inactivity. Never let a child eat while watching television—or see you doing it!

Fast food chains everywhere make junk food attractive to children and parents with toy surprises, playgrounds, waving balloon figures, drive-through lanes, and cheap and ready short orders. Busy parents fall for them, especially when a child wears them down with begging and whining. Take-out dinners are easy. No preparation, and no clean-up for tired parents. Of course it is harder to make dinner at home, and harder still to get the children to help. But how much more rewarding!

Children find fast food restaurants exciting. Tomato ketchup on the hamburger. Lots of little packages to open up, spill—and throw away. Doughnuts and buns, sweet carbonated drinks, fries with salt (and often added sugar!), and plenty of fat all become an unhealthy habit. Very soon, a child won't eat unless she can have sweetened drinks, salty foods with ketchup, and desserts— all readily available, and all advertised on TV at every break.

Once a child's taste buds have become accustomed to these overpowering tastes, you may have lost her to these foods. These foods and others like them are likely to lead to cavities, obesity, and diabetes. They fill a child up with "empty calories" and do not offer the vitamins and other nutrients children need for the healthy development of their brains and bodies. Healthy foods—with less salt, less sugar, fewer and healthier fats, and more varied tastes and textures—won't stand a chance when in direct competition with junk food.

Don't make a big deal about it, but stock your kitchen with appealing foods that are also nutritious, not junk food. Your children will probably get plenty of junk food at their friends' homes, and even in some schools where the big soda pop and fast food companies have bought their way in. Simply say, "Chips and soda are fine once in a while, but we don't need them every day." Say much more, and you'll only pique your child's interest in these forbidden fruits. There is no harm in an occasional ice cream cone or handful of chips. The trouble with junk food is that it can all too easily take over and turn into a junk food diet. This can certainly be avoided since there are plenty of healthy recipes—in cookbooks and on the Internet— for easy-to-make, affordable, and most important of all, tasty snacks and meals to appeal to children.

We are in the midst of an obesity epidemic in the United States, and childhood diabetes, too, is on the rise. Inactivity is one reason, but junk food is also one of the main causes.

Very busy families who rely on take-out dinners should know that some are healthier than others: salad, fruit salads,

---

Healthy Snacks to Keep in the House

- Fresh fruit
- Raisins (for children over 3) and other dried fruit
- Nuts (for children over 4)
- Whole grain crackers, bagels, rolls
- Unsweetened fruit juice (100 percent fruit juice, not fruit drinks)
- Cheese
- Yogurt
- Applesauce (avoid added sugar)
- Dry cereal (choose ones with low sugar content)
- Homemade cookies with wholesome ingredients like oatmeal, nuts, raisins, and modest amounts of fat and sugar

certain ethnic foods such as Chinese dishes with vegetables and steamed rice (brown is better than white), and Greek specialties such as stuffed grape leaves, pita bread and hummus, or "wraps" with lean meat, chopped vegetables, and cheese.

Lead, Lead Poisoning, and Pica

Lead Poisoning

Lead poisoning is a very serious disorder because it can interfere with brain development in fetuses and in children in the first 5 years of life, and lead to hyperactivity, poor attention, and other learning and behavioral problems. It can also cause anemia (a weakening or shortage of red blood cells). Before it causes any symptoms, an elevated lead level can be detected in cord blood at birth and later with blood tests done at routine pediatric appointments. If you live in an old house, you should be sure your pediatrician checks your child's blood for elevated lead levels and anemia. Flakes of paint and dust containing lead peel off onto windows, sills, and the floor. When a crawling 8-month-old baby finds that lead paint chips taste sweet, she'll quickly learn to search for and savor them.

Take some chips to the doctor with you so that they can be tested too. You can then find out if you need to strip your house of the offending paint or plaster. Early symptoms of lead poisoning include irritability, sleep and appetite problems, and constipation. Later, vomiting and headaches occur, along with stomach aches, clumsiness, weakness, confusion, seizures, and finally even coma. Long before this, effective treatment for lead poisoning is available—the sooner the better.

Lead poisoning is all too common and can be prevented by protecting young children from any exposure to lead—in old lead water pipes, lead paint, house dust from lead paint, soil contaminated with lead (from lead paint and other sources), and cookware containing lead. If you live in an older home, have your water tested for lead. Lead paint should be removed from homes in which young children live—before they arrive, or else when the family is staying elsewhere, and never while they are living there. The stripping and chipping of paint and wood will leave chips and dust particles of lead all around. In some towns and cities, financial assistance is available for lead paint removal. Check with your local public health department.

Pica

As soon as a child finds that she can use thumb and index finger to pick up tiny objects (pincer grasp), at around 8 months, she must be watched more carefully. Now she can pick up and eat any tiny object she finds on the floor. A baby will eat hair, wool objects, paper, pieces of string, flakes of paint and plaster chips, clay, dirt, tacks—any object small enough to fit in her mouth and swallow. Fortunately, she's likely to spit out objects that have no taste or are inedible, but parents can't count on that.

Pica is the medical term for frequent and repeated attempts to eat non-edible materials. In some cases, for example, prolonged, repetitive eating of clay or dirt, it appears that an iron or zinc deficiency causes the behavior. Although it is normal for infants to explore their world by putting all kinds of objects in their mouths, this behavior should subside by about age 4 or 5.

If a child's hunger for foreign objects persists and is a problem, try bits of food to distract her. If these do not work, consult a behavioral clinic at a children's hospital for ways to treat pica with other positive reinforcement techniques.

Mealtimes as Family Time

Children thrive on structure. A chance to share breakfast and dinner with parents gives them a beginning and an end to the day. When parents are busy and must leave the child all day, this becomes even more important. In this stressed world, regular mealtime rituals say, "Your world is as safe as we can make it. We are all together and we will face the world together."

Parents who must be away all day can make the evening meal a time for reunion. "What did you do today? I missed you!" Make it a fun time, when everyone gets a chance to share their experiences. No comments on food or how much a child is eating or not eating.

Understood rules can become part of the ritual. "Everyone has an opportunity to share what we have. No special meals. If you don't like what we're having, I hope you'll like the next meal better." Parents are bound to regret it if each child comes to expect that her tastes will be catered to with a food prepared just for her. Also, make it clear that "once you begin to play with food, or to tease about it, your meal is finished."

Many families find it challenging to get to the breakfast table together. Plan to wake up 15 or 20 minutes earlier, so that you can spend that time with your family to start off the day. To help your child get to the breakfast table on time, lay out her clothes the night before. Put a glass of orange juice beside her bed. She can drink it *before* she gets up to help her get going. Many children have such low blood sugar levels that they feel grumpy. After the juice boosts her blood sugar, she may feel better and act better. Then you can help her prepare to separate before going off to childcare or school with a breakfast together. A well-balanced breakfast (nonsugary cereals, with milk and fruit, or eggs with toast, for example) is, of course, the most important solution for early morning low blood sugar. But it also can become a shared family time when plans for the day can be made. As breakfast ends, talk about when you'll be together again, at the end of the day.

Children who are started early in setting the table, clearing it, and helping with the dishes will feel that they are part of their family's work together. On Sunday morning let them help decide what to eat for breakfast, and let them share in the preparation. The more they can choose and help with the meal, the more it can become a family celebration. "You chose this for all of us. Thank you!"

Milk and Milk Allergies

Breast milk is ideal for babies. Replicating it has become the goal of formula manufacturers. In an effort to improve on breast milk, iron has been added to "fortified formulas." Some babies cannot tolerate this added iron, and it may contribute to colicky stomach pains. (Babies get by with the iron from their own red blood cell stores until they are 4 to 6 months old. Then they may need more iron than is usually present in breast milk. Breast milk contains small but variable amounts of iron. But babies on breast milk may be more likely to absorb iron more easily than babies on formula.)

Rarely, a baby may react to breast milk. This is usually due to some food in the mother's diet. The problem is likely to disappear when the mother can identify and eliminate the culprit.

A few babies are unable to digest lactose, the sugar in cow's milk. This is referred to as *lactose intolerance*—it's not an allergy. Some babies with lactose intolerance will be able to digest this milk sugar later on, after their intestines have had time to mature or to heal from an infection that has temporarily caused it. Lactose intolerance should not cause a rash or trouble breathing, since it is not an allergic reaction. Usually, the main symptom is diarrhea, along with stomach pain.

A small minority of babies are allergic to cow's milk protein and cannot tolerate the cow's milk in formulas. This is called *milk protein allergy.* Repeated spitting up, stomach pains, diarrhea, rashes, and even trouble breathing are signs that the baby is allergic to milk protein and needs a substitute. Your child's pediatrician can help you select one.

If the switch does calm down your baby's symptoms, you'll know not to give her milk or milk products until much later—the second or third year. Then, watch for any allergic response to recur. Meanwhile, your pediatrician should make sure that the substitute formula covers her protein, calcium, fat, and vitamin requirements throughout her infant years. Some infants who are allergic to milk will also be allergic to soy-based formula. There are substitutes for soy milk if your baby is allergic to it.

An infant with a milk protein allergy may be more likely to develop other food allergies, so go slow; during the first year, avoid foods that are most likely to cause allergies: eggs (especially egg whites), nuts, soy, oranges and other citrus fruits, chocolate, shellfish, and corn and wheat products.

Signs of Milk Protein Allergy

- Frequent spitting up, vomiting
- Signs of abdominal pain (or colic), such as frequent crying, especially after feedings, irritability, difficulty soothing
- Diarrhea, bloody stools—there are, of course, other causes for this that your doctor will also want to check for
- Scaly skin rash (atopic dermatitis) usually appears later, by 6 months of age
- Hives (urticaria)—big, raised, red bumps over the skin
- Trouble breathing, swelling (especially of mouth and throat), lethargy—these can be signs of a serious allergic reaction that requires emergency attention from a doctor

What to Do If You Suspect a Milk Allergy

1. *If your child is having trouble breathing, call for emergency help.*
2. Talk to your doctor about the signs of milk allergy you are concerned about. She or he will want to sort out a milk protein allergy from lactose intolerance, since the treatments are different.
3. Ask your doctor about stopping cow's milk formula and trying a soy-based formula instead. However, some infants allergic to milk proteins will also be allergic to soy-based formula. A lactose-intolerant baby can be switched to a lactose-free formula.
4. If you want to be sure that cow's milk was indeed the problem, talk to your doctor about slowly starting her back on very small amounts of cow's milk again—after she's recovered from her earlier troubles. If the same symptoms recur, you'll know that the cow's milk was the culprit. But *don't try this* if your baby had any serious allergic reaction symptoms, such as eczema, trouble breathing, swelling, or lethargy.
5. As they get older, some babies will be able to digest cow's milk products comfortably. But check with your doctor before reintroducing cow's milk products.

Nutritional Needs

Children's nutritional needs change as they grow. There are a few peak periods of rapid growth. The first year of life is a time of greater growth than any other in childhood: weight increases by 200 percent, length by 55 percent, and head circumference by 40 percent! Puberty and early adolescence are next, when the rate of growth is again astounding. It is not surprising, then, that children's food requirements are highest during these periods.

In the first week or two of life, newborns are busy adjusting to their new environment, and they lose a little weight. After the first week or so, though, they'll get going again. Of course, babies may not seem to eat a lot compared with older children, but they certainly feed more often, and in relation to their weight, they actually eat far more than older children. One of the reasons why food struggles are so common after the first year is that children's rate of growth starts slowing down, and parents may not realize that their child is often less hungry and may not need to eat quite as much.

There is a limit to this slowdown though. Although growth has slowed by 1 year of age, activity levels are on the rise. The toddler's high-energy crawling, standing, and walking also require calories as fuel.

No parent fails to recognize the next burst in food consumption, in early adolescence. Grocery bills go up, refrigerators burst at the seams, and children seem to shoot up overnight.

For most children, hunger is the best guide to their food requirements. This can be thrown off if they have unbalanced diets, with too much of one kind of nutrient (for example, soda and other sweets or saturated fats) and not enough of the others. These nutrients may fill them up without supporting their growth. If you are uncertain about your child's food requirements or fear that your child's growth is not adequate, consult her pediatrician. She or he will check your child's weight, height, and head circumference, may look for medical causes for failure to grow, and may refer you to a dietitian to help identify your child's food requirements for healthy growth.

Of course, children need a healthy balance of proteins (for example, fish, chicken, beans, tofu, and red meat), fats (for example, vegetable oils as well as the fat in meats, dairy products, and even fish and grains), and carbohydrates (for example, whole grain breads, pasta, rice, certain vegetables, fruits, and dairy products).

In the current Food Pyramid prepared by the U.S. Department of Agriculture, the following amounts of various types of foods are recommended for children of ages 2 to 6 every day.

- Grains (bread, pasta, rice, etc.), 6 servings
- Vegetables, 3 servings
- Fruit, 2 servings
- Milk, 2 servings (16 ounces total, each day)
- Protein (meat, beans, eggs, etc.), 2 servings
- Fats and sweets, sparingly

Serving sizes will change with the age of the child. A typical serving size for a 4-year-old might be half a cup of milk, an egg or 1–2 ounces of lean meat, one-third of a cup of rice or cereal, half a cup of salad, and half a banana or apple.

Children also need a healthy balance of vitamins, minerals, and trace elements. The best way to accomplish this is by offering children a wide variety of different foods. The necessary balance changes as children grow. In infancy, vitamin D and iron are more likely to be lacking. In later childhood, calcium is often insufficient. There are many helpful books that supply detailed information about a child's nutritional needs as she develops. (See *Books for Parents* in Bibliography.) Check with your pediatrician about the balance of your children's diet. For many children, multivitamin supplements are unnecessary, and some vitamins and minerals can even be dangerous if given in excess.

Overweight Children

Americans are facing an epidemic of overweight children today—an estimated 20 percent of all children are obese. A child is considered obese if she is 20 percent above her normal weight for height and age. Obesity can also be defined as weight levels that put well-being and health at risk.

Overweight children suffer from being teased and from the resulting poor self-esteem. They may also avoid or have trouble succeeding in sports. This condition can also lead to medical problems in childhood (high blood pressure and cholesterol, sleep apnea, and joint problems, among others). It also can increase the risk of these and other disorders in adulthood (for example, cancer, diabetes, and heart disease). Childhood obesity is a major risk factor for obesity in adulthood.

Genetics plays a role in obesity, so any child with overweight parents is at risk. But in our country, children are also put at risk by fast foods and processed foods, full of unhealthy fats, sugars, and salt in oversized portions, nutritionally "empty" calories that don't supply a balance of necessary nutrients. Healthier foods, with more fiber and protein, are not the ones being pushed in television advertisements and fast food joints, and they may be more expensive. Sadly, our country's poorest children are most at risk.

Added to our unhealthy diet is our couch potato culture. Television, video and computer games, and the Internet take time away from physical activity. As fields and forests are taken over by malls and unsafe housing developments, and child-safe sidewalks are replaced by freeways, more children are kept indoors, in front of the TV.

For some children, there may be additional factors in weight gain. Some children may turn to food for comfort and soothing, particularly if they never learned other ways of comforting themselves. Some children may never have learned to pay attention to hunger and fullness cues. We'd expect this to be more common in children who never learn to enjoy sitting down for relaxed mealtimes with their families, but instead have meals in front of the TV and snack and graze all day. Children are more likely to learn to handle their appetites when mealtimes (and snacks) occur at regular, predictable times that have a beginning, middle, and end—such as salad to start with, then the main course, and finally dessert. If you are concerned about your child's weight, let your pediatrician know—*early*. In any case, your pediatrician should be monitoring your child's growth (weight and height) at each routine preventive visit. Overweight children under 2 years of age are likely to be obese later, as older children. Uncommon medical causes of weight gain, including hormone abnormalities, need to be considered. Depression can also lead to excess weight gain.

Many children gain a little weight just before entering puberty. Unless the gain is excessive, it should not be cause for concern. Children this age are often very sensitive about their appearance, and a parent's reaction to bodily changes can be very upsetting. Don't comment on it. If you are concerned, discretely ask for your pediatrician's advice at your child's routine visit. If your child is concerned, listen to her, let her know that you understand that it bothers her, but let her know that this is a normal change and that you are not worried.

What to Do When a
Child Truly Is Overweight

After age 2 or 3, you can switch from whole milk products to low-fat ones. Skip fried foods. Substitute lower-fat sources of protein such as chicken, fish, and beans for red meat when you can. But even low-fat foods can have lots of calories—in the form of sugars and carbohydrates—and cause weight gain. (Examples are juices, sugary cereals, and candy.) Switch from juice—especially bottled juices high in sugar, and calories—to water. Fresh fruits and vegetables, which are high in fiber and vitamins, are healthier for overweight children than many processed or packaged foods. Whole grain breads and pasta, brown rice, and similar foods are an improvement over foods containing refined flour.

Weight gain is inevitable when the amount of calories a child eats is greater than the amount she burns off. Attention to an overweight child's diet must be balanced by an increase in physical activity. Walk or ride a bike (always wear helmets) with your child instead of driving to school or to do errands whenever possible. Have your child help out with physical chores around the house and garden. Encourage her to participate in school and after-school sports or dancing, although you may need to work with her to help her learn basic skills that she may have missed out on if she's been hiding from sports. Be sure none of this becomes a burden or a struggle. Let her participate in choosing her favorite fitness activity. The focus should be on health, *not* appearance. Try to make all of this as matter-of-fact as possible, or still better, fun!

Your child won't be interested if she feels hurt by any suggestion from you that she is overweight. Instead of starting with your concerns, listen to her—children at school tease her, she can't run as fast as she wants, she's embarrassed by having to wear "husky-size" clothes, and so on. When she comes to you with concerns like these, don't tell her that she's overweight. Instead ask her, "Would you like to try to work on this?" If she says no, then simply say, "If you ever do, there are some things that can help. Just let me know when you're ready." If she isn't ready, there is no point in pushing her—it won't work. Meanwhile, keep listening, limit junk foods and TV and computer time, and try to set examples of healthy eating and physical activity yourself. These measures should be for all family members, so as not to focus negatively on the overweight child.

But if your child says she is ready, ask her, "Would you like a few ideas about foods that you'll enjoy eating that will help you feel healthier? Would you like to know which foods might be better to try to cut back on?" Assure her that you know she needs to eat, and that she shouldn't have to go without eating when she's hungry. As you begin to help her, continue to make sure that this is her initiative, not yours. A parent might even suggest, "We could find an exercise program for you, if you'd like." Examples are children's fitness programs at the local YMCA or Boy's and Girl's Club. Some children may be more comfortable working on this with a professional rather than with a family member.

If you can help your child discover her own motivation to take on and overcome this challenge, she's far more likely to succeed. Be careful. If she feels that this is your issue and not hers, she'll be at risk of even more overeating—a vicious cycle indeed.

Picky Eaters

Some children have especially sensitive taste buds, which can interfere with eating ordinary foods that parents offer. A parent might think, "All the other babies eat table foods if they are cut up for them. Mine won't. Is she just testing me, or is there a real reason?" I would advise that you simply avoid the foods and the textures that she may be particularly sensitive to. Instead, use alternatives with similar nutritional value. Forget the foods she's resisting until she is older. There's no point in setting up resistance in her as she learns to feed herself.

Many children react to their parents' pressure (direct or subtle) to eat by becoming picky eaters. Being picky in the second and third years is their way of testing their parents. "I won't eat that. Give me a peanut butter sandwich," a picky eater might say. Anything to resist the food parents offer. But parents who try to please the child are giving in to the "game" and won't set up the boundaries she may need. Instead of rushing to prepare something different, a parent might say, "This is what we're having for dinner tonight." The child's demands for other reasonably healthy foods can be handled by responding, "What a good idea! That can be for another meal." But don't change the menu on the spot for a picky eater. She may not eat the new choices you offer either, and she'll know now how to keep you jumping.

The best way to prevent picky eating before it starts is for parents to make a regular habit of offering a broad variety of food choices without forcing any of them on the child. Over time, even picky children who are exposed to a wide range of foods—without pressure—are more likely to develop a taste for them.

Premature and Fragile Babies and Feeding

There are many kinds of fragile babies. They may be premature, or they may be full term but subtly underfed by the placenta during pregnancy. Or they may have been delivered with difficulty and need to reorganize and recover. The term also includes babies who were born with a range of medical conditions, some hereditary, some arising during pregnancy, some without explanation.

A premature or otherwise fragile baby must quickly be evaluated and understood. As she recovers from the first major stress—birth—she must muster her strength to adjust to her new world. How easily overwhelmed she'll be by all the new adjustments—to independent breathing, circulation, and temperature control, to new, demanding noises and lights, to her own reflex motor responses no longer contained by the uterus, and to getting the nutrients and fluids she needs in a whole new way. How can a fragile infant manage so many adjustments in such a short time?

The miracle of birth and survival places enormous demands on parents as well. Parents will grieve about the baby they might have had and struggle to face their fears about this baby's future. "Will she survive? Will she be damaged for life? Do I want her to live if she is impaired? If she lives, can I learn to manage with her?" Any parent of a fragile baby will be faced with these questions, and then with the challenge of nurturing the baby after discharge from the hospital's neonatal intensive care unit (NICU). A parent may be too overwhelmed to request the help and understanding necessary to adjust to the baby. I would urge parents to visit their baby in the NICU as often as possible and to learn from her nurses how to protect her, handle her, and feed her. As she recovers and makes her adjustment, so will you.

Feeding Difficulties

Many of these babies will encounter difficulties in feeding. Difficulty in swallowing—due to neurological damage or developmental delays impairing swallowing mechanics, gastroesophageal reflux after feedings, hypersensitivity of the intestinal system leading to colic and irritability, hypersensitivity of the nervous system to auditory, tactile, visual, and kinesthetic stimuli—all require special handling at feeding times. All of these need to be understood by new, frightened parents *before* discharge. The opportunity to soothe and heal these fragile babies' disorganized nervous systems can be enormous if parents can model on nurses, doctors, and others trained to handle these babies with the special care they need. It is a parent's right to ask for such help. (See *Resources.*)

Patience and careful observation of the baby's behavior will be a great help. A premature or otherwise fragile baby must reorganize slowly. Many different systems—circulatory and respiratory systems, nervous system and sensory apparatus, and gastrointestinal tract—will be entwined in this recovery. These will need to become integrated in order for the baby to begin to thrive.

This process will demand patience and understanding from parents. They must be ready to reduce stimulation (such as noise, lights, even handling) for the baby. Yet their hunger for her to recover and to "catch up" is likely to press them to push her to eat, eat, eat. This will very likely work the wrong way, for example, by overloading a sensitive GI tract, resulting in regurgitation or diarrhea.

Premature and low-birth-weight babies face a double challenge. On the one hand, they need far more nutrients relative to their weight than full-term babies do. On the other, their digestive systems are often not yet well developed enough to handle these amounts.

Formulas

Special formulas are available for premature infants, and specialized dietitians in the hospital will help decide which formula to use, whether it needs to be diluted, and how much and how often it can be given. Sometimes premature infants must be fed with feeding tubes or with intravenous fluids containing the nutrients they need until they can suck on their own and their digestive systems are mature enough to handle formula.

Breastfeeding

It is certainly possible, though a challenge, to give premature infants breast milk. They may initially be too weak to suckle at the breast, so a mother who wants to breastfeed will need to express milk—while at the NICU or when at home. A mother's milk, even when the pregnancy has ended too soon, contains an ideal balance of proteins as well as antibodies to help protect the baby from infections. A specialized dietitian can mix the mother's milk with the extra nutrients that a premature infant requires.

The mother of a premature infant needs and deserves extra support—from family, NICU staff, and a lactation consultant if she wants one. Carrying a baby skin-to-skin, between the mother's breasts or in a sling on her chest, is called "kangaroo care." It stimulates the mother's milk supply and helps her to feel close to her baby. It's good for the baby too.

Parents will need to observe and to adapt to their baby's individual situation. For example, their baby may tolerate feedings only every 3 hours rather than every 4 hours. A slower feeding in a quiet, darkened room may be necessary at first. Later, parents can gradually add stimulation, watching for signs that the baby has had enough—spitting up, hiccups, or a bowel movement. Her face may darken, as her body arches away and her color changes, which are all signals that she is overwhelmed. If she is overstimulated, she's likely to vomit up all the food she's managed to get down. She needs protection from too many sights and sounds and motion if her progress is to continue, although this can be difficult in a busy household.

Parents who have been through a difficult adjustment to a premature or fragile baby are very likely to hover over the baby. They find it difficult to allow her to go through the normal, inevitable "touchpoints" as she gets older without tremendous anxiety. At touchpoints when backslides in the area of feeding might be expected, parents are bound to worry and press the child to eat. This may hold her back from learning to feed herself when she is able to. Such parents may have trouble accepting her defiance, especially when food is involved. They are bound to stifle such bids for independence, urging, "Just try this, darling!" A baby, especially a once fragile baby, needs many chances to feel successful, to be able to say to herself, "I did it myself!" The child will always win in a struggle over food, and this is the wrong place for parents to set up a conflict. I urge parents of a fragile baby not to hover, but instead to encourage the child toward self-sufficiency and to seek help if you aren't sure how to proceed. Don't push food on your child, for you can only lose.

Rewards, Punishments, and Food

Don't use either rewards or punishments to handle a child's challenging eating behavior. Also don't use food as rewards or punishments for any other disciplinary issue. When food is used in this way, it can lose its meaning as an element of survival and a source of pleasure, and meals can lose their meaning as a time for positive interactions. Serious eating problems can be the sad result. For example, when a parent says, "No dessert if you misbehave," a child who feels she needs to punish herself for some deep-seated reason may see self-starvation as a way to do this. (Or else it may just make dessert all the more alluring.) When a parent says "you can have an extra helping if you're really good," a child who is hungry for more love or approval may turn to overeating to find it.

Your role is to decide on what and how much food to offer a child. You can set up a pleasant atmosphere at meal times. But you can't force food into a child's mouth, and you can't make her swallow it. Inevitably, it will be up to the child to decide what, when, and how much she will eat. If you try bribes or punishments to force a child to eat, you'll fail.

Even if a child has learned to enjoy her meals and her feedings with you in the first year, she is still likely to become defiant and start testing in the second year. But you can get through it if you're ready for it, and can plan to *enjoy* it with her. Your sense of humor will be your best defense.

Let her test you. It's fairly simple to be sure she receives her nutritional requirements (see *Nutritional Needs* in this chapter) throughout the second and third years. Meals should be times for warmth and and fun—not ordeals.

Desserts

Should desserts be saved for rewarding a child who has eaten well, and withheld from one who has not? No. Dessert is a conclusion, a way to end a meal—not a reward. Making dessert a reward makes it more desirable than the other food a child must learn to eat! Offer the whole family the same kind of dessert, so that it does not become a reward or a punishment.

Some candy-like, processed food desserts are overpoweringly enticing. They, along with the TV commercials that make them even more irresistible, can push children over the edge—into relentless, demanding tantrums. If desserts become a focus of struggles, they should be traded for more nutritious ones—fruits, yogurt, ice cream (low-fat if weight is an issue), and the like. But don't present healthier food choices as a punishment! If heavy, sugary, fatty desserts like sundaes, rich cake and cookies, and puddings are never introduced or are reserved for special occasions (such as birthday parties), you'll spare yourself and your child a lot of anguish. She may make you feel as if you've deprived her terribly. Don't worry. You haven't, and she'll get over it.

Rumination

Rumination is an uncommon disorder in which an infant, usually between 3 and 12 months of age, regurgitates food to chew on after a feeding. (It also occurs in some older children.) She makes sucking or chewing movements. She may shove her fingers down her throat to help her regurgitate the food. She may arch her back to help push food up.

Parents of such babies are frantic. Their anxiety adds to the baby's underlying problem and the baby fails to gain weight, or may even lose weight. A baby with these symptoms needs to be checked on by a specialist (a pediatric gastroenterologist) in order to be sure that there is not an underlying medical illness. Such conditions may include pyloric or lower esophageal stenosis, hiatal or diaphragmatic hernia, gastroesophageal reflux (see *Spitting Up, Gastroesophageal Reflux, and Pyloric Stenosis*), or a gastrointestinal infection, among others.

Meanwhile, babies who ruminate for no medical reason may be trying to tell you that they are either under- or overstimulated at feeding (and other) times. Try to see whether you and she can find ways of making feeding time more satisfying. You may need to feed her in a less stimulating environment if you have several other, noisy children. You may need to rock and sing gently to her *before* you start feeding her. You may need to talk lovingly after a feeding, when she is propped up to avoid regurgitation.

If rumination continues, seek help from your pediatrician (who, after checking for medical causes, may refer you to a behavioral specialist experienced in handling rumination). Your anxiety, understandable though it is, may only add to the problem, and an expert can help you handle it so that you can help your child overcome this upsetting disorder.

School Lunches

When parents prepare a lunch "from home" for a child to take to school, food takes on an additional meaning for the child: It becomes a connection to parents, a private moment to remember them and feel close to them when she is at school. I can still remember the oozy peanut butter sandwiches and the occasional piece of leftover fried chicken that I found in my lunch box as a schoolboy in Waco, Texas. This food was a tie to home and to the parents who had sent me off. The lump in my throat caused by our separation would always subside when I ate my wing of chicken.

Every sandwich, every apple, every piece of celery carries a symbolic message to the child. And you can put in a special note from time to time: "Have fun at school today!" or "Remember our plans for this weekend!"

Preparing a child's lunch box is also an opportunity to let her make choices about her food, and even to let her do some of the work to get it ready. She will be even more excited when she opens up her lunch box at school to see the dessert she picked out, the extra napkins she scrunched in. Of course, it takes more time to prepare lunch than to give your child money to buy it at school. But if you and your child do it together—for example, after supper, when you can divert leftovers for this purpose—this can be a special time for you to be together!

If your child does eat the school meals, find out what is being served. Are there healthy choices or only fast food? Also, do children stock up at vending machines with sweets and soda and boycott real food at the cafeteria? Sometimes parents need to organize and speak up if the school lunches are unhealthy, if fast food chains have bought their way in, or if soda pop is freely available.

Spitting Up, Gastroesophageal Reflux, and Pyloric Stenosis

Spitting Up

Spitting up is often confused with vomiting and gastroesophageal reflux. Vomiting pushes food forcefully out of the mouth, while spitting up just causes it to dribble. Most babies spit up or dribble small amounts of undigested liquid (breast milk or formula) now and then, especially after a feeding or with bubbling. After spitting up, a baby is unlikely to cry. The adult who'd just picked her up and now has fresh spittle on her shoulder is more likely to be distressed than the baby. But when a baby vomits, larger amounts of partly digested food or formula make a bigger mess and a baby cries out in pain.

Vomiting that goes on for just a day or so is most likely to be due to a gastrointestinal infection or stomach flu, especially if the baby also has a fever. The biggest challenge will be to help the baby hold in enough fluids to protect against dehydration. (See *Illnesses and Eating.*) Vomiting or spitting up large amounts after feeding that goes on for longer, though, may be a sign of a number of different medical problems, including gastroesophageal reflux (GER). Call your doctor to be sure you get help in determining the cause as soon as possible.

Many babies who gulp down their milk are likely to spit up after feedings. It may seem as if they have GER, when some of these babies may just need to slow down and be helped to swallow smaller amounts at a time. Prop them at a 30-degree angle afterward and gravity will help. Some babies spit up small amounts until 7 or 9 months of age.

Gastroesophageal Reflux

Gastroesophageal reflux (GER) is a condition that can occur in a baby's first year when the ring-shaped muscle (sphincter) at the top of the stomach has not yet grown strong enough to keep food in the stomach from flowing back up into the esophagus. As a result, food, usually a liquid feeding, that has made its way down the esophagus and into the stomach comes back up again. The baby vomits or spits up large amounts after most feedings—often all over you. The food or liquid may appear partially digested. When a baby has a weak gastroesophageal sphincter, the food that comes back up into the esophagus contains acid from the stomach. The stomach acid mixed in with the food hurts—and the baby cries after each meal.

Be sure to let your pediatrician know that you are concerned about your baby's spitting up or vomiting, and describe your observations about what helps too. When GER is the diagnosis, medications can sometimes cut down on stomach acid and help the stomach move its contents down "the right way."

Severe GER interferes with weight gain and growth and requires urgent medical attention. It can also occasionally cause ulcers in the esophagus because of the stomach acid, or damage to the lungs when stomach contents come back up and then go

---

Signs of Gastroesophageal Reflux (GER)

- Frequent vomiting up of large amounts with feedings
- Signs of pain with feedings, including crying, or arching of the back
- Coughing or choking with feedings
- Fussiness, irritability after feedings
- Refusal to feed—arching, turning away
- Bloody vomit or stools
- Failure to gain weight, or weight loss

Although gastroesophageal reflux is more common, your doctor will also check for other causes of these symptoms, especially if they are severe.

down "the wrong way," through the trachea to the lungs. The resulting pain and trouble breathing can be so distressing to a baby that food refusal and failure to thrive may develop, adding a new layer of problems. Ear and lung infections are also more likely to develop when a baby has GER.

What to Do for Gastroesophageal Reflux (GER)

- Bubble and burp your baby after each feeding. (See *Bubbling and Burping* in Chapter Two.)
- Check your baby's position during and after feedings. Be sure she is propped at a 30 degree angle during feedings and for at least 30 minutes after feedings—longer if needed.
- Don't sit her straight up in a baby chair, as she'll just slump forward, defeating the purpose.
- Give your baby smaller feedings more often. Keep cutting back the amount of each feed until the spitting up is better. Try using an ounce or two less at a feeding to see if it helps. But be sure you feed her more often, often enough so that she still gets the same total amount of breast milk or formula every day.
- Some doctors recommend thickening formula with cereal "to help it stay down." Be sure that it is not so thick that it clumps up, clogging the nipple or requiring too much of the baby's energy to suck down. Some studies, though, have failed to show that this makes a difference.
- Your doctor may prescribe medication to neutralize the stomach acid and to help the stomach empty feedings into the intestine rather than sending them back up the wrong way. These should be considered especially if reflux is severe, such as when it interferes with breathing or growth.

If severe reflux and pain persist, a specialist (a pediatric gastroenterologist) should evaluate the baby. Milk allergy may be a cause of the vomiting. Your baby may need diagnostic testing to determine the extent of her problem and to help in deciding on a more intensive treatment. Fewer than 10 percent of children with true GER require surgical intervention, but your baby's physician should certainly help you with strategies to cut down on reflux vomiting.

If you put your baby down on her stomach (stay with her to be sure she stays awake in this position) or on her back with her head elevated, plan to play quiet games with her to keep her from getting agitated and pushing the stomach contents up. This is likely to work for most babies with GER, and the sphincter will mature and strengthen with time.

Infants should begin to outgrow this condition by 7 months. Further improvement will occur by 9 months, when she is likely to keep herself upright during and after feedings on her own. By 2 years of age, gastroesophageal reflux symptoms have usually stopped for good.

Pyloric Stenosis

Projectile vomiting—vomiting so forceful that digested food shoots out at a distance from the baby's body—can be a sign of a more serious problem, pyloric stenosis. Pyloric stenosis is a condition in which the opening of the lower end of the stomach into the duodenum (the beginning of the intestine) is too tight to let food through. This leads to projectile vomiting, sending partially digested food out 1 to 4 feet from the baby's body about 10 or 15 minutes after feedings. This kind of vomiting usually begins when a baby is 3 to 6 weeks old. If projectile vomiting occurs several times at this age, you should contact your baby's doctor promptly.

Pyloric stenosis is uncommon, and it occurs more often in boys than girls. This disorder interferes with weight gain and growth, so if it is diagnosed, your pediatrician will recommend a straightforward and effective type of surgery. Projectile vomiting should always be taken seriously and checked out. (See also *Rumination.*)

Table Manners

Table manners are learned from modeling on older children and adults. But don't expect them to emerge until age 4 or 5. Still, parents should plan on modeling—right from the start—the manners they'd like their children to imitate. A parent who says, "Thank you," when handed half a soggy cookie is already encouraging the child to see that such a response is an expectation. However, when asked to say "thank you," a 2-year-old cannot be expected to respond except in imitation.

A 3-year-old may try out "thank you," "hello grandma," or using a spoon or fork at the table, but she's just as likely to tease you by dropping them. She may say "thank you" one time, but "ugh" the next. Don't expect your child to be consistent. Patient repetition is the key. If you expect too much and get irritated, you will make manners into a bother or a burden instead of a way for a child to show respect, learn her place—and others'—in the world, and win people over.

By age 4, a child begins to realize and value her effect on the world. By 4 or 5, she is aware that her manners do matter and will get her the approval of those around her. She begins to try them out. She uses her napkin on rare occasions. She tries to cut food with her knife. She uses her fork, although maybe only once her fingers have become sticky, or because it is more fun to spear a carrot than to spoon it. Manners are on their way.

By age 6 and over, I would expect manners. Repetition and patience will still be needed, though. You may even let your child know what you expect ahead of time. For example, "When we're all having dinner with our friends, you'll need to remember to ask to be excused before you leave the table." But pressure can take away the incentive your child may have to become socially successful *on her own.*

Television and Eating Habits

Any parent who feeds a child in front of the television is setting up problems for the future. "But it distracts her, and she eats better," a parent may protest. Maybe so, but food and TV are best kept separate.

Television is too overstimulating. A child who needs some distraction while she is eating will do far better to be distracted by conversation with you. A child needs to eat in a quiet and relaxed atmosphere so that she can learn to pay attention to her

Keeping Television and Meals Separate

- Making television (or junk foods) entirely off limits may only work temporarily.
- Longer-range solutions, such as sports, games, and other more appealing alternatives to TV, should be encouraged.
- Children who have not been raised on television are bound to find most of the shows and commercials far less interesting than the other activities they've grown accustomed to.
- Seek the child's help in the kitchen or setting the table instead of having the TV do the baby-sitting while you prepare supper.
- If you must have a TV, have only one in the house. Maybe a poor quality one, with lousy reception, that isn't too much fun to watch! Put it in a room where the family doesn't spend much time—never in the kitchen or the child's bedroom.
- Never eat and watch TV at the same time. Eating should be limited to mealtimes and scheduled snacks, and should be allowed only while sitting down at the kitchen or dining room table. You'll be thrilled at how much easier it is to keep your house clean—though your dog may not be!
- Don't be rigid about television. Instead of forbidding it altogether (which may work for some families, but may backfire for others), pick out a special show or video to watch together.

body when it tells her she is hungry or she is full. A child who does not know when she is full, and just keeps on eating as long as her favorite show is on, is at risk of becoming overweight.

Television, even without food added to it, is our biggest competitor for our children's hearts and minds. Add food to TV time, and you'll make it even harder to pry your child away.

If children get used to meals with television, they're bound to start snacking while they watch too. Grazing, outside of regular snack times, can interfere with eating at meals, and also contribute to obesity.

Time spent in front of the TV takes away from time for physical activity, another risk factor for obesity. Television ads pressure children to pop in junk food while they watch. TV is one contributor to a problem of epidemic proportions in the United States—childhood obesity and later related medical problems such as high blood pressure and diabetes. Passive TV watching, coupled with high-calorie, low-nutrition junk food and disrupted mealtimes, is setting up a serious health threat to our children. Don't let them eat and watch TV at the same time!

Mealtimes in front of the TV take away from time for your family to be together. Lose these opportunities for communication now, and your children may be more likely to shut you out when they are adolescents. Make mealtimes as pleasant and enjoyable as you can. Less emphasis on the amount eaten and more on being together will help in the long run. (See *Overweight Children* and *Mealtimes as Family Time.*)

Throwing Food

Nearly all 9- to 12-month-old babies throw food if you give them more than they want. Or even if you don't. Put a big tarpaulin under your baby's high chair, or invite the dog in, or feed your baby in an empty bathtub (where it doesn't matter).

It helps to put only two table bits at a time in front of her. If she's hungry and is only given such a small amount, she's more likely to put them in her mouth. When she swallows them, put two more in front of her. Meanwhile, don't hover over her. If you do, you may unintentionally encourage her to rebel. When she begins to play with her bits of food or throws them over her chair, put her down. Say, as matter-of-factly as you can, "That's it—until the next meal."

Don't overdo your reaction to food refusal or throwing. A quiet, firm statement carries more meaning. A child will learn quickly that if she wants her food, she'd better eat it instead of throwing it. Let her know that throwing is a clear message that she's through.

Vegetarians

For much of the first year of life, most infants rely primarily on breast milk or formula for their nutritional needs. As they grow, toddlers and children being raised as vegetarians can continue to get all of the nutrients they need without eating meat. But special attention will be needed to ensure that their diet contains adequate amounts of certain nutrients—for example, protein, iron, calcium, and vitamin B_{12}.

Good sources of protein include dairy products and eggs (for vegetarians who include those in their diet), whole grains, and soy-based foods. Iron from meat is more readily absorbed than iron from plant sources, but children can absorb adequate amounts of iron from whole grain foods, iron-fortified cereals, legumes (chickpeas, soybeans, black beans, and others), some green leafy vegetables (like spinach), peas, and dried fruits. If dairy products are not included in a child's diet, calcium can be obtained from calcium-fortified juices, cereals, and soy and rice milks. Some beans, nuts, and green leafy vegetables also contain calcium. Vitamin B_{12} is found only in animal products. If eggs and dairy products are excluded, vitamin B_{12}–fortified foods or supplements are necessary. (See *Resources.*)

Vitamins and Minerals

According to many physicians, many foods and formulas are so well fortified with vitamins and minerals that extra vitamins are not necessary when children eat well-balanced diets. But the whimsies of older babies and toddlers as they refuse one food after another may make vitamin supplementation necessary. When parents can count on supplements to fill in important, though hopefully temporary gaps in a child's diet, it becomes easier to stay out of food struggles.

Vitamin supplements can be a small price to pay for your comfort in knowing that your child's nutritional needs are covered. Using a multivitamin supplement to cover temporary refusal of vegetables is a sure, simple way to avoid this refusal from becoming a struggle and a bigger, longer-lasting problem. It's worth it!

Your pediatrician may recommend vitamin drops (for example, vitamin D and perhaps iron) in infancy, which are easiest to give while the baby is positioned and ready for her milk. Chewable vitamins later let her participate more actively. But be careful: She is likely to be eager for the tasty chewable. Don't leave them around. A toddler can overdose on chewable vitamins "because they're so good." Keep chewable vitamins tightly capped, locked up, and out of her reach.

Babies and children need a balance of the full range of vitamins, minerals, and trace elements. A different regular amount of each is needed. There is no better or worse vitamin or mineral, and more is not necessarily better. While some vitamins given in excess will simply be excreted by healthy children, others can be dangerous to give in large amounts. A deficiency of any vitamin, mineral, or trace element can lead to physical symptoms—ask your doctor about your child's diet if you are concerned that something is missing. For a few vitamins and minerals, ensuring adequate supplies in the diet may be difficult without supplements. Among these are iron, calcium, vitamin D, and for vegetarians, vitamin B_{12}.

Iron

Up until 4 to 6 months, a baby usually has adequate iron stores because she is still relying on iron transferred from her mother's body before birth. But by 4 to 6 months, a baby will need more iron, sometimes more than breast milk and nonfortified formulas contain. Breastfed babies may absorb iron more easily than formula-fed babies, but many formulas are fortified with iron. Ask your doctor if your baby needs iron supplements.

Without enough iron, a baby or young child may develop anemia (weak or deficient red blood cells). It now appears that iron deficiency anemia may sometimes even interfere with healthy brain development and contribute to learning disabilities.

Calcium

Calcium is important for healthy bone development. Fortunately for most infants and young children, there is a good supply of it in milk. Later, though, children often drink less milk than they need. Dairy products—cheese, yogurt, and ice cream—are also good sources, and calcium is sometimes added to orange juice. Calcium absorption by bones is critical throughout childhood and peaks during adolescence. Adolescents need about 1,200 mg of calcium per day in order to protect against osteoporosis (weakened, brittle bones) later in life. Yet, most—by some estimates, 60 percent of adolescent boys and 80 percent of adolescent girls—are not getting enough calcium. This is a major concern, since adult bones will not absorb as much calcium as children's do.

Vitamin D

Calcium absorption depends on adequate amounts of vitamin D. A good source of vitamin D is vitamin D–fortified milk, and vitamin D is sometimes added to orange juice too. (Solid dairy products, such as cheese, though, do not contain added vitamin D.) The American Academy of Pediatrics now recommends a total intake of 200 International Units of vitamin D per day for babies, starting in the first 2 months of life and continuing throughout childhood and adolescence. Many doctors believe that 400 International Units per day is needed. While most formulas are fortified with vitamin D, breast milk may not contain enough. Ask your baby's doctor if she should have a vitamin D supplement, at least until she is weaned and drinking a cup and a half or more of vitamin D–fortified formula or milk every day. But don't overdo the supplements, since too much vitamin D is harmful.

Vitamin D deficiency, leading to poor calcium absorption and weak bones, is more common in regions where there is less sunlight and in darker-skinned people. This is because sunlight absorbed through the skin actually activates vitamin D. Without enough sunlight exposure, there may not be enough activated vitamin D to ensure that bones absorb the calcium they need to be strong. In young children, a calcium or vitamin D deficiency can lead to severely bowed legs. This is even more of a concern now that doctors are recommending that children and adults (including breastfeeding mothers) limit their sun exposure to avoid skin cancer. Ask your doctor about vitamin D supplements for your baby, especially if you and your baby have darker skin, live in a climate with long winters and lots of gray days, or have little vitamin D in your diets. (See also *Nutritional Needs.*)

Bibliography

Books for Children

Baer, Edith, and Bjorkman, Steve. *This Is the Way We Eat Our Lunch: A Book About Children Around the World.* New York: Scholastic Books, 1995.

Cole, Joanna, and Relf, Patricia. *The Magic School Bus Gets Eaten: A Book About Food Chains.* New York: Scholastic Books, 1999.

Dr. Seuss. *Green Eggs and Ham.* New York: Random House, 1960.

Dr. Seuss. *Scrambled Eggs Super.* New York: Random House, 1953.

Books for Parents

Abrams, Richard S. *Will It Hurt the Baby? The Safe Use of Medications During Pregnancy and Breastfeeding.* Reading, MA: Addison-Wesley, 1990.

Brazelton, T. B. *Touchpoints: Your Child's Emotional and Behavioral Development.* Cambridge, MA: Perseus Publishing, 1992.

Brazelton, T. B., and Sparrow, J. D. *Discipline: The Brazelton Way.* Cambridge: Perseus Publishing, 2003.

Brazelton, T. B., and Sparrow, J. D. *Sleep: The Brazelton Way.* Cambridge: Perseus Publishing, 2003.

Brazelton, T. B., and Sparrow, J. D. *Toilet Training: The Brazelton Way.* Cambridge: Da Capo Press, 2004.

Brazelton, T. B., and Sparrow, J. D. *Touchpoints 3–6: Your Child's Emotional and Behavioral Development.* Cambridge: Perseus Publishing, 2001.

Curtis, Glade B., and Schuler, Judith. *Your Pregnancy for the Father-to-Be.* Cambridge: Perseus Publishing, 2003.

Feinbloom, Richard I. *Pregnancy, Birth, and the Early Months: The Thinking Woman's Guide.* Cambridge: Perseus Publishing, 2001.

Hirschmann, Jane R., and Zaphirpoulos, Lela. *Preventing Childhood Eating Problems: A Practical, Positive Approach to Raising Children Free of Food and Weight Conflicts.* Carlsbad, CA: Gurze Books, 1993.

Leach, Penelope. *Your Baby and Child: From Birth to Age Five.* New York: Knopf, 1997.

Mason, Diane, and Ingersoll, Diane. *Breastfeeding and the Working Mother.* New York: St. Martin's Press, 1986.

Pruett, Kyle. *Fatherneed: Why Father Care Is as Essential as Mother Care for Your Child.* New York: Free Press, 2000.

Rosenberg, Ronald, Greening, Deborah, and Windell, James. *Conquering Postpartum Depression: A Proven Plan for Recovery.* Cambridge: Perseus Publishing, 2003.

Schlosser, Eric. *Fast Food Nation: The Dark Side of the All-American Meal.* New York: Harper Collins, 2002.

Tamborlane, William V. (ed.). *The Yale Guide to Children's Nutrition.* New Haven: Yale University Press, 1997.

Thirion, Marie. *L'allaitement.* Paris: Albin Michel, 1994.

Woolf, Alan, Kenna, Margaret, and Shane, Howard, eds. *Children's Hospital Guide to Your Child's Health and Development.* Cambridge: Perseus Publishing, 2001.

References for Professionals

American Academy of Pediatrics. "Pediatric Food Allergy." *Pediatrics* supplement, Vol. 111, No. 6, June 2003.

Benoit, D. "Failure to Thrive and Feeding Disorders," in Zeanah, C. H. (ed.), *Handbook of Infant Mental Health.* New York: Guilford, 1993.

Cashdan, E. "A Sensitive Period for Learning About Food." *Human Nature* 5: 279–291, 1994.

Chang, Tien-Lan. "Gastroesophageal Reflux," in Dershowitz, R. (ed.), *Ambulatory Pediatric Care,* 3rd ed. New York: Crown-Raven, 1998.

Dixon, Suzanne, and Stein, Martin (eds.). *Encounters with Children.* St. Louis: C.V. Mosby, 2000.

Gartner, Lawrence M., and Greer, Frank R. "Prevention of Rickets and Vitamin D Deficiency: New Guidelines for Vitamin D Intake—An American Academy of Pediatrics Clinical Report." Pediatrics 111(4): 908–910, April 2003.

Hallberg Leif, Hoppe Michael, Anderson Maria, and Hulthen Lena. "The Role of Meat to Improve the Critical Iron Balance During Weaning." *Pediatrics* 111(4): 864–870, April 2003.

Kaiser Study. *Kids and Media at the New Millenium.* 1-800-656-4533.

Kessler, D. B., and Dawson, P. (eds.). *Failure to Thrive and Pediatric Undernutrition: A Transdisciplinary Approach.* Baltimore: Paul H. Brookes Publishing, 1999.

Law, Karen L., Stroud, Laura R., LaGasse, Linda L., Niaura, Raymond, Liu, Jing, and Lester, Barry M. "Smoking During Pregnancy and Newborn Neurobehavior." *Pediatrics* 111(6): 1318–1323, June 2003.

Ludwig, David S. "The Glycemic Index: Physiological Mechanisms Relating to Obesity, Diabetes, and Cardiovascular Disease." *Journal of the American Medical Association* 287(18): 2415–2423, May 8, 2002.

National Research Council and Institute of Medicine. Shonkoff, Jack P., and Phillips, Deborah A. (eds.). *From Neurons to Neighborhoods: The Science of Early Childhood Development.* Washington, DC: National Academy Press, 2000.

Pipes, Peggy L., and Trahms, Cristine M. *Nutrition in Infancy and Childhood.* St. Louis: Mosby, 1993.

Radzyminski, Sharon. "The Effect of Ultra Low Dose Epidural Analgesia on Newborn Breastfeeding Behaviors." in Journal of Obstetric, Gynecologic, and Neonatal Nursing 32(3): 322–331, May-June 2003.

Ramsay, Mary. "Feeding Disorder and Failure to Thrive," in Minde, Klaus (ed.), *Child and Adolescent Psychiatric Clinics of North America: Infant Psychiatry,* Vol 4, No. 5, July 1995, pp. 605–616.

Ransjo-Arvidson Anna-Berit, Matthiesen Ann-Sofi, Lilja Gunilla, Nissen Eva, Widstrom Ann-Marie, Uvnas-Moberg Kerstin. "Maternal Analgesia During Labor Disturbs Newborn Behavior: Effects on Breastfeeding, Temperature, and Crying." *Birth* 28(1): 5–12, March 2001.

Samour, Patricia Queen, Helm, Kathy King, and Lang, Carol E. *Handbook of Pediatric Nutrition.* Gaithersburg, MD: Aspen Publications, 1999.

Sepkoski, C., Lester, B., Ostheimer, G. and Brazelton, T. B. "The Effect of Maternal Anesthesia on Neonatal Behavior During the First Month." *Development and Medical Child Neurology* 34(2): 1072–1080, December 1992.

Sparrow, J. D. "Adolescent Eating Disorders: in Dershowitz, R. (ed.), *Ambulatory Pediatric Care,* 3rd ed. New York: Crown-Raven, 1998.

Walker, W. Allan, and Watkins, John B. *Nutrition in Pediatrics—Basic Science and Clinical Application.* Hamilton (Ontario), BC: Decker, 1996.

Wenzl, Tobias G., Schneider, Sabine, Scheel, Frank, Silny, Jiri, Heimann, Gerhahrd, and Skopnik, Heino. "Effects of Thickened Feeding on Gastro-Esophageal Reflux in Infants: A Placebo-Controlled Crossover Study Using Intraluminal Impedance—Abstract." *Pediatrics* 111(4): 875, April 2003.

Woolston, J. L. (ed.). "Eating and Growth Disorders," in *Child and Adolescent Psychiatric Clinics of North America.* Philadelphia: W. B. Saunders, January 1993.

Videotapes

Brazelton, T. B., et al. *Discipline* (I Am Your Child Foundation)
www.iamyourchild.org

Brazelton, T. B., et al. *Touchpoints* (videotape volumes 1–3)
Available through:
The Brazelton Touchpoints Center
1295 Boylston Street
Suite 320
Boston, MA 02115

Resources

American Academy of Allergy, Asthma, and Immunology
611 E. Wells Street
Milwaukee, WI 53202
(800) 822-2762 or (414) 272-6071
Fax: (414) 272-6070
www.aaaai.org

American Academy of Pediatrics
141 Northwest Point Boulevard
Elk Grove Village, IL 60007-1098
(847) 434-4000
Fax: (847) 434-8000
www.aap.org

American Dietetic Association
120 S. Riverside Plaza
Suite 2000
Chicago, IL 60606-6995
(800) 877-1600
www.eatright.org
hotline@eatright.org

American Pseudo-Obstruction and
Hirschsprung's Disease Society
158 Pleasant Street
North Andover, MA 01845-2797
(978) 685-4477
Fax: (978) 685-4488
www.tiac.net/users.aphs

Asthma and Allergy Foundation of America
1125 15th Street, N.W., Suite 502
Washington, DC 20005
(800) 7-ASTHMA, (800) 727-8462, (202) 466-7643
www.aafa.org

Celiac Disease Foundation
13251 Ventura Boulevard, #1
Studio City, CA 91604-1838
(818) 990-2354
Fax: (818) 990-2374
cdf@celiac.org

Center for Science in the Public Interest
1875 Connecticut Avenue, N.W.
Suite 300
Washington, DC 20009
(202) 332-9110
www.cspinet.org
This organization publishes *Nutrition Action*, a magazine about healthy
    food choices, food safety, and current nutrition controversies.

Cystic Fibrosis Foundation
6931 Arlington Road
Bethesda, MD 20814
(800) 344-4823
www.cff.org

Depression After Delivery
www.depressionafterdelivery.org

Eating Disorders Awareness and Prevention, Inc.
603 Stewart Street
Suite 803
Seattle, WA 98101
(800) 931-2237 (information and referral hotline)
(206) 382-3587
Fax: (206) 829-8501
www.edap.org

The Food Allergy Network
4744 Holly Avenue
Fairfax, VA 22030-5647
(703) 691-3179
Fax: (703) 691-2713

International Lactation Consultants Association
4101 Lake Boone Trail, Suite 201
Raleigh, NC 27607
(919) 787-5181
Fax: (919) 787-4916
www.ilca.org

La Leche League International
1400 North Meacham Road
Schaumburg, IL 60173
(800) LALECHE (breastfeeding warmline)
(847) 519-0035
www.lalecheleague.org

Medic Alert Foundation International
2323 Colorado Avenue
Turlock, CA 95382
(888) 633-4298, (800) 432-5378
www.medicalert.org

National Alliance for Breastfeeding Advocacy
http://hometown.aol.com/marshalact/Naba/home.html

National Association of Anorexia Nervosa
and Associated Disorders (ANAD)
Box 7
Highland Park, IL 60035
(847) 831-3438 (hotline)
Fax: (847) 433-4632
www.anad.org

National Digestive Diseases Information Clearinghouse
2 Information Way
Bethesda, MD 20892-3570
(800) 891-5389
Fax: (301) 907-8906
digestive.niddk.nih.gov
niddc@info.niddk.nih.gov

National Institute of Allergy and Infectious Diseases
31 Center Drive, MSC 2520
Building 31, Room 7A50
Bethesda, MD 20892-2520
(301) 496-5717
Fax: (301) 402-0120
www.niaid.nih.gov

National Institute of Diabetes and Digestive and Kidney Diseases
2 Information Way
Bethesda, MD 20892-3570
(301) 654-3810
Fax: (301) 907-8906
www.niddk.nih.gov

National Safe Kids Campaign
1301 Pennsylvania Avenue, N.W.
Suite 1000
Washington, DC 20004
(800) 441-1888
(202) 662-0600
Fax: (202) 393-2072
www.safekids.org

Newborn Individualized Developmental
Care and Assessment Program
Attn: Heidelise Als, PhD
Children's Hospital
300 Longwood Avenue
Boston, MA 02115
(617) 355-8249
Fax: (617) 277-0199
www.nidcap.com/nicap

Tufts University Health and Nutrition Letter
10 High Street
Suite 706
Boston, MA 02110
Healthletter@tufts.edu
www.healthletter.tufts.edu

Tufts Nutrition Navigator (a guide to and rating of nutrition websites)
http://navigator.tufts.edu

The Vegetarian Resource Group
Box 1463
Baltimore, MD 21203
(410) 366-8343
http://vrg.org

U.S. Consumer Product Safety Commission
Washington, DC 20207-0001
(800) 638-2772 (consumer hotline)
www.cpsc.gov

Zero to Three: National Center for Infants, Toddlers, and Families
734 15th Street, N.W.
Suite 1000
Washington, DC 20005
(202) 638-1144
www.zerotothree.org

Hotlines

The American Academy of Allergy and Immunology
(800) 822-2762

The American Academy of Pediatrics
(800) 433-9016

Eating Disorders Awareness and Prevention, Inc.
(800) 931-2237

National Association of Anorexia Nervosa
Associated Disorders (ANAD)
(847) 831-3438

The National Center for Nutrition and Dietetics
(800) 366-1655

Index

About the Authors

T. Berry Brazelton, M.D., founder of the Child Development Unit at Children's Hospital Boston, is Clinical Professor of Pediatrics Emeritus at Harvard Medical School. His many important and popular books include the internationally best-selling *Touchpoints* and *Infants and Mothers*. A practicing pediatrician for over forty-five years, Dr. Brazelton has also created the Brazelton Foundation (www.brazeltonfoundation.org) to support child development training for healthcare and educational professionals around the world.

Joshua D. Sparrow, M.D., is Assistant Professor of Psychiatry at Harvard Medical School and Special Initiatives Director at the Brazelton Touchpoints Center. He is the co-author, with Dr. Brazelton, of *Touchpoints Three to Six, Calming Your Fussy Baby: The Brazelton Way, Sleep: The Brazelton Way, Discipline: The Brazelton Way,* and *Toilet Training: The Brazelton Way.*